NUTRITIONAL IMPACTS
on WOMEN
Throughout Life
with Emphasis on
Reproduction

77–78–79–80–81–82—10–9–8–7–6–5–4–3–2–1

Cover and text designed by Alice J. Sellers

DRUG DOSAGE

The authors and publisher have exerted every effort to ensure that drug selection and dosage set forth in this text are in accord with current recommendations and practice at the time of publication. However, in view of ongoing research, changes in government regulations, and the constant flow of information relating to drug therapy and drug reactions, the reader is urged to check the package insert for each drug for any change in indications and dosage and for added warnings and precautions. This is particularly important when the recommended agent is a new and/or infrequently employed drug.

Library of Congress Cataloging in Publication Data
Main entry under title:

Nutritional impacts on women.

  Includes index.
  Bibliography: p.
  1. Pregnancy—Nutritional aspects. 2. Mothers—
Nutrition. 3. Women—Nutrition. I. Moghissi, Kamran S.
II. Evans, Tommy Nicholas, 1922–
RG559.N87   612.6   76–43296
ISBN 0–06–141793–9

Contents

LIST OF CONTRIBUTORS   ix

PREFACE   xiii

FOREWORD   xv

1
Nutritional Ages of Woman
William J. Darby   1

2
Physiologic Basis of Nutritional Needs During Pregnancy and Lactation
Angus M. Thomson, Frank E. Hytten   10

3
The Implications of Undernutrition During Pubescence and Adolescence on Fertility
Samuel M. Wishik   23

4
Nutrition in the Adolescent
William J. McGanity   30

5
Effects of Maternal Dietary Restrictions During Pregnancy on Fetal Growth and Maternal–Fetal Exchange in the Mammalian Species
Pedro Rosso   49

6
Factors in Intrauterine Impoverishment
John A. Churchill   69

7
Amino Acid Sources for the Fetus
Roy M. Pitkin   75

viii

8
Relationship of Maternal Amino Acids and Proteins to Infant Growth and Mental Development
Kamran S. Moghissi   **86**

9
The Effect of Maternal Alcohol Ingestion During Pregnancy on Offspring
Eileen M. Ouellette, Henry L. Rosett   **107**

10
Carbohydrate Metabolism—Some Aspects of Glycosuria
Tom Lind   **121**

11
Maternal Nutrition—Its Effects on Infant Growth and Development and Birthspacing
Hernan L. Delgado, Aaron Lechtig, Charles Yarbrough, Reynaldo Martorell, Robert E. Klein, Marc Irwin   **133**

12
Relationship of Nutrition to Lactation and Newborn Development
Lloyd J. Filer, Jr.   **151**

13
Effect of Oral Contraceptives on Micronutrients and Changes in Trace Elements Due to Pregnancy
Ananda S. Prasad, Kamran S. Moghissi, Kai Y. Lei, Donald Oberleas, Joan C. Stryker   **160**

14
Hormonal Contraception and Nutrition
Mark A. Belsey   **189**

15
Nutrition in Menopausal and Postmenopausal Women
E. Neige Todhunter   **201**

EPILOGUE
Clinical Application of Nutrition in Perinatal Practice
Ronald A. Chez   **220**

INDEX   **225**

List of Contributors

Mark A. Belsey, M.D.
CHAPTER 14
Medical Officer, Human Reproduction Unit, World Health Organization, Geneva, Switzerland

Ronald A. Chez, M.D.
EPILOGUE
Chief, Pregnancy Research Branch, National Institute of Child Health and Human Development, Bethesda, Maryland

John A. Churchill
CHAPTER 6
Professor, Department of Neurology, Wayne State University School of Medicine, Detroit, Michigan

William J. Darby, M.D., Ph.D.
CHAPTER 1
President, The Nutrition Foundation, Inc., New York, New York; Professor of Nutrition, Department of Biochemistry, Vanderbilt University, Nashville, Tennessee

Hernan L. Delgado, M.D.
CHAPTER 11
Scientist, Division of Human Development, Institute of Nutrition of Central America and Panama, Guatemala City, Guatemala

Lloyd J. Filer, Jr., M.D., Ph.D.
CHAPTER 12
Professor, Department of Pediatrics, University of Iowa College of Medicine, Iowa City, Iowa

Frank E. Hytten, M.D., Ph.D., F.R.C.O.G.
CHAPTER 2
Head, Division of Perinatal Medicine, Clinical Research Center, Harrow, England

Marc Irwin, Ph.D.
CHAPTER 11
Scientist, Division of Human Development, Institute of Nutrition of Central America and Panama, Guatemala City, Guatemala

Robert E. Klein, Ph.D.
CHAPTER 11
Director, Division of Human Development, Institute of Nutrition of Central America and Panama, Guatemala City, Guatemala

Aaron Lechtig, M.D.
CHAPTER 11
Scientist, Division of Human Development, Institute of Nutrition of Central America and Panama, Guatemala City, Guatemala

Kai Y. Lei, Ph.D.
CHAPTER 13
Assistant Professor, Interdisciplinary Nutrition Program, Department of Home Economics, Mississippi State University, Mississippi State, Mississippi

Tom Lind, M.B., B.S., Ph.D., M.R.C.O.G.
CHAPTER 10
Consultant Obstetrician and Gynecologist, Scientific Staff, Medical Research Council Reproduction and Growth Unit, Princess Mary Maternity Hospital, Newcastle Upon Tyne, England

William J. McGanity, M.D., F.R.C.S.(C)
CHAPTER 4
Professor and Chairman, Department of Obstetrics and Gynecology, University of Texas Medical Branch, Galveston, Texas

Reynaldo Martorell, Ph.D.
CHAPTER 11
Scientist, Division of Human Development, Institute of Nutrition of Central America and Panama, Guatemala City, Guatemala

Kamran S. Moghissi, M.D., F.A.C.O.G., F.A.C.S.
CHAPTER 8, 13
Professor of Gynecology and Obstetrics; Chief, Division of Reproductive Biology, Wayne State University School of Medicine, C.S. Mott Center for Human Growth and Development, Detroit, Michigan

Donald Oberleas, Ph.D.
CHAPTER 13
Research Chemist, Research Service, Veterans Administration Hospital, Allen Park; Associate Professor of Biochemistry in Medicine, Department of Medicine, Wayne State University School of Medicine, Detroit, Michigan

Eileen M. Ouellette, M.D.
CHAPTER 9
Associate Professor, Department of Pediatrics and Neurology, Boston University School of Medicine, and Boston City Hospital, Boston, Massachusetts

Roy M. Pitkin, M.D.
CHAPTER 7
Professor, Department of Obstetrics and Gynecology, University of Iowa College of Medicine, Iowa City, Iowa

Ananda S. Prasad, M.D., Ph.D.
CHAPTER 13
Professor of Medicine; Director, Division of Hematology, Department of Medicine, Wayne State University School of Medicine, Detroit; Staff Physician and Acting Chief of Staff, Department of Medical Research, Veterans Administration Hospital, Allen Park, Michigan

Henry L. Rosett, M.D.
CHAPTER 9
Associate Professor of Psychiatry, Department of Psychiatry, Boston University School of Medicine; Assisting Physician, Department of Psychiatry, Boston City Hospital, Boston, Massachusetts

Pedro Rosso, M.D.
CHAPTER 5
Assistant Professor of Pediatrics and Obstetrics and Gynecology, Institute of Human Nutrition, College of Physicians and Surgeons, Columbia University, New York, New York

Joan C. Stryker, M.D.
CHAPTER 13
Associate Professor, Department of Gynecology and Obstetrics, Wayne State University School of Medicine; Chief, Outpatient Department, Hutzel Hospital, Detroit, Michigan

Angus M. Thomson, M.B., Ch.B.
CHAPTER 2
Director, Medical Research Council Reproduction and Growth Unit, Princess Mary Maternity Hospital, Newcastle Upon Tyne, England

E. Neige Todhunter, Ph.D.
CHAPTER 15
Visiting Professor of Nutrition, Vanderbilt University School of Medicine, Nashville, Tennessee; Professor of Nutrition, School of Home Economics, University of Alabama, Tuscaloosa, Alabama

Samuel M. Wishik, M.D.
CHAPTER 3
Professor Emeritus, Public Health Administration, School of Public Health; Consultant, Center for Population and Family Health, Columbia University, New York, New York

Charles Yarbrough
CHAPTER 11
Scientist, Division of Human Development, Institute of Nutrition of Central America and Panama, Guatemala City, Guatemala

Preface

During the past few years several monographs on nutrition have been published, but none addressed to the nutritional needs of women or to the nutrition required for optimal reproductive performance. This book represents a new approach to this important area of medicine—a composite of information derived from many different disciplines concerned with human reproduction and the impact of nutrition on it. The chapters of this book have been prepared by experienced clinicians, scientists, and investigators in different areas of human nutrition with one thing in common: their desire to explore how best to improve the health of women from early childhood through reproductive years and past menopause.

This book clearly delineates the important role of nutrition in normal and abnormal human reproduction, presenting a broad range of epidemiologic, biochemical, and related considerations. The dietary requirements of women during their reproductive years are specifically delineated. The effect of nutritional deficiencies during pregnancy and parturition is reviewed in detail, clarifying relationships between nutrition and birth defects including subsequent motor and mental deficits. Attempts have been made to include in each chapter older standard concepts as well as more recent studies. Several chapters include original information hitherto unpublished.

The editors hope that this book will supplement the knowledge of physicians providing care for women of all ages. It should prove particularly useful to medical students, graduate students in obstetrics, gynecology, and pediatrics, as well as basic scientists engaged in nutritional research and clinicians who care for patients with reproductive problems. It is hoped that these contributions from several countries will intensify interest and stimulate research in this long-neglected area. We will feel amply rewarded if better understanding of nutritional principles by clinicians will in some measure improve the health and well being of their patients.

We wish to express our appreciation to Marlene Visconti-Taipalus for editorial assistance and to Harper and Row for their encouragement and helpful collaboration in publishing this volume.

K.S.M.
T.N.E.

Foreword

Clinical nutrition is not usually regarded to be a glamorous medical discipline. It is taught inadequately in most medical schools and poorly applied by most clinicians. This is deplorable since the consequences of inadequate nutrition are among the most important health problems. Conservative estimates are that 25 percent of the world population suffers from starvation and another 25 percent receives substandard nutrition. It is believed the world population will reach 6.5 to 7 billion by the year 2000. Clearly, despite technologic and agrarian advances, food production cannot keep pace with the increasing demands.

While developed, industrially advanced and wealthier nations are less prone to suffer from inadequate food supply or nutritional deprivation, it is naive to believe that they can be totally spared in view of the burgeoning population and our finite nutritional resources. It has been repeatedly shown that in many large urban and some rural areas of the United States, the most prosperous and agriculturally advanced country in the world, malnutrition is prevalent and results in many health problems.

As physicians and teachers we have a well-defined task before us. We must revise medical school curricula and teach nutrition as a major course rather than as an appendix to biochemistry and physiology. With the scientific tools at our disposal, we must investigate and explore the health consequences of malnutrition and undernutrition, expose damaging food fadism and instruct our patients about the health consequences of improper nutrition.

As gynecologists and obstetricians we have a heavier burden since we are directly or indirectly involved in the health care of women for most of their lives. Our teaching of nutrition in gynecology-obstetrics has not been superior to that of other disciplines. Many of our colleagues are confused as to what is adequate nutrition for an adolescent girl, a parturient, a lactating mother or a menopausal woman.

Simultaneous control of our rapidly expanding population and rapid improvement in human nutrition must be the most vital objectives of all concerned with the preservation and improvement of the quality of life.

NUTRITIONAL IMPACTS
on WOMEN

Chapter 1

Nutritional Ages of Woman

William J. Darby

This monograph concerns the relationship of nutrition to woman's health, the preconceptional nutriture of the mother, the dependence of the fetus and infant on the maternal organism, the subsequent physiologic eras of development and reproduction, and the postreproductive years of the aging woman. The data and interpretations presented are derived from somewhat fragmentary, albeit extensive, investigations dealing with the more distinct, nonconnected aspects of the nutrition of women. Some of these studies made in the 1940s and early 1950s covered the relationship of nutrition during pregnancy to the outcome of pregnancy and the health of the infant. They include the extensive investigations of Hoobler and Mack in Detroit; Scrimshaw and collaborators in Rochester; Ebbs, Tisdall, and coworkers in Toronto; Burke *et al.* in Boston; Dieckmann *et al.* in Chicago; and the Vanderbilt Cooperative Group in Nashville. The physiologic studies by Professor Hytten and his collaborators (6) represent still another aspect of this broad problem. This approach is illustrated by the chapters in this monograph authored by Thomson and Lind. These and related investigations are summarized in a report of the Committee on Maternal Nutrition of the Food and Nutrition Board (7) which provides an extensive bibliography of the literature up to 1970. A prior monograph of the Food and Nutrition Board prepared by Toverud, Stearns, and Macy (15) provides an excellent historical perspective on earlier studies of maternal nutrition and child health.

During the past 25 years, a broader spectrum of workers with everwidening interests and expanded approaches have introduced considerations more comprehensive than those of preceding investigators. Improved, more sensitive techniques have enabled the study of nutrients that previously could not be quantitated. Current journal articles carry exciting findings, such as those from the Human Nutrition Laboratory of the United States Department of Agriculture-Agricultural Research Service on the striking effect of trace element nutriture on pregnancy. An example is the effect of maternal zinc deficiency (8) on the reduction of fetal brain cell size, the complement of DNA, RNA, protein, and lipid in the liver, as well as the reduction of incorporation of thymidine into hepatic DNA. Of startling significance, sociologically, are reports of increased aggressiveness (5) in female offspring of zinc-deficient mothers (*i.e.*, rat dams). Male offspring of these zinc-deficient dams exhibit impaired avoidance conditioning and decreased tolerance to stress. The intensive interest manifest today in the nutrition and metabolism of trace elements (12) was accelerated by human

1

zinc deficiency studies reported by Prasad, Sandstead, and others of the Vanderbilt–NAMRU-3 (U.S. Naval Medical Research Unit Number 3) research group working in Cairo in the 1950s and 1960s.

Society's awareness of the importance of maintaining nutrition and of societal responsibility for assuring that food needs be fulfilled has resulted in new concern for improved understanding of the nutritional needs of the older population. Accordingly, there exists a new interest in the need to define the nutritional requirements of menopausal and postmenopausal woman. Such definition of requirements demands a greater understanding of both the physiologic and the social factors affecting women during the latter part of their life. Similarly, concern for one's exposure to environmental and nonfood influences has directed attention to the effects of smoking, alcohol ingestion, chronic drug therapy, and the use of metabolic regulators such as oral contraceptives. An awareness of the problems of the developing world and a better understanding of the limitations on the rate and type of social development are stimulating the reexamination of many accepted Western diet patterns and attitudes, including those surrounding the practices of breast-feeding and artificial feeding of infants. All of these influences are reflected in the content of this volume.

AGES OF WOMAN, AS MODIFIED FROM SHAKESPEARE

An appropriate classification of the nutritional ages of woman may be provided by taking minor liberties with a brief quotation from Shakespeare's *As You Like It*—*i.e.,* changing and modernizing the Bard's enumeration of the ages of man to conform to the subject of woman.

> *All the world's a stage,*
> *And all men and women merely players:*
> *They have their exits and their entrances;*
> *And one woman in her time plays many parts,*
> *Her acts being five ages.*
> At first, the infant,
> *Mewling and puking in the nurse's arms.*
> And then the whining school-girl, *with her satchel*
> *And shining morning face, creeping like snail*
> *Unwillingly to school.* And then the lover,
> *Sighing like furnace, to a woeful ballad*
> *Played on her lover's lute.* And then the wife,
> *Her fair round belly with growing fetus lin'd,*
> *With work severe and dress of maternal cut.*
> And then the lean and slippered pantaloon,
> *With spectacles on nose and T.V. on side . . .*
>
> *With apologies to William Shakespeare*

And as "one woman in her time plays many parts"—from infant to "lean and slippered pantaloon"—her nutritional needs change . . . from age to age, and even within an age. Let us briefly overview these nutritional ages.

"AT FIRST, THE INFANT"

During the first year of life, the body weight increases some 7 kg and the body's composition changes from 11 to 14.6% protein (13). According to Fomon (4), the increment in body protein is 3.5 g/day during the first 4 months of life and 3.1 g/day during the next 8 months. By the age of 4 years, body protein reaches the adult level of 18–19%. At birth, energy allowances are at a level of 120 kcal/kg/day and decrease to 100 kcal/kg by the end of the first year.

The corresponding need for lesser nutrients is such that food of high nutrient density, *i.e.,* high concentration of essential nutrients per 100 kilocalorie of energy, must be supplied to avoid deficiencies. Two striking consequences of this principle may be cited. One is the widespread occurrence in the developing world of *kwashiorkor,* with its manifestation of protein deficiency and evidence of associated deficits of other nutrients (vitamin A, folic acid, tocopherol, and zinc, for example). Another consequence more familiar to us in the United States is the appearance of *iron deficiency anemia* as the infant approaches the end of its first year of life, a deficiency that results from the low nutrient density of iron in milk, a deficit that now, fortunately, is widely recognized and compensated for in practice.

Social Conditions and Infant Nutrition

The requirement of the infant and young child for sustenance of high nutrient density cannot be separated from its social implications. These are well considered in scholarly perspective by Aykroyd (1), the first Director of the Nutrition Division of the Food and Agriculture Organization of the United Nations (FAO), and are worthy of mention here.

Aykroyd quotes Sir John Simon (14), a great pioneer in public health, who, in 1861, wrote a description of the then existing social conditions and their consequences for infant feeding and health in England:

Factory women soon return to labour after their confinement. The longest time mentioned as the average period of the absence from work in consequence of child-bearing was five or six weeks; many women among the highest class of operatives in Birmingham acknowledged to having generally returned to work as early as eight or ten days after confinement. The mother's health suffers in consequence of this early return to labour . . . and the influence on the health and mortality of children is most baneful. . . . Mothers employed in factories are, save during the dinner hours, absent from home all day long, and the care of their infants during their absence is entrusted either to young children, to hired girls, sometimes not more than eight or ten years of age, or perhaps more commonly to elderly women, who eke out a livelihood by taking infants to nurse. . . . Pap, made of bread and water, and sweetened with sugar or treacle, is the sort of nourishment usually given during the mother's absence, even to infants of a very tender age. . . . Illness is the natural consequence of this unnatural mode of feeding infants. . . . Children who are healthy at birth rapidly dwindle under this system of mismanagement, fall into bad health, and become uneasy, restless and fractious. . . . Abundant proof of the large mortality among the children of female factory workers was obtained.[14]

In 1906, Newman (9) estimated that "hand-fed" infants had a lower chance of survival than did breast-fed infants by a mortality ratio of 3:1. These infants deprived of breast milk were given various substances as the principal article of diet: fresh milk diluted to different degrees; condensed milk, especially skimmed, sweetened, condensed milk; "starchy" foods such as bread, biscuits, oatmeal, and arrowroot; "patent" foods, usually consisting of malted starch, sugar, and some dried milk. All these foods and food mixtures were associated with high infant mortality. The worst were sweetened, skimmed, condensed milk and the starchy foods; diluted fresh milk gave somewhat better prospects of survival, but was usually lethal enough because of pollution and ignorance on the part of mothers of the proper degree of dilution. The "patent" foods varied in their effects; some were rather better than others. The quantities of substitutes for breast milk given to hand-fed infants were often insufficient so that undernutrition as well as malnutrition resulted.

His survey of infant mortality convinced Newman of the extreme importance of suitable infant feeding. "It is not everything," he said, "but a greater factor than any other thing. . . . Even the domestic and social conditions are reducible to terms of nourishment."

Aykroyd (1) notes the similarities of the conditions described in England 50 to 70 years ago with those that pertain to developing countries today: high infant mortality rate, predominating percentage of deaths in the postnatal period, high mortality in the second year of life, weaning diarrhea, measles as a serious disease, and unavailability of suitable infant foods other than breast milk.

He then observes:

Whereas there may be a few discrepancies, it is reasonable to suppose that something like the complex of malnutrition and infection that we now call protein-calorie malnutrition [PCM] was prevalent in the affluent countries until recently, with disastrous effects on infant and child health. Clinical observations and vital statistics show that it has almost entirely disappeared from these countries. Its disappearance has been hastened by the establishment and development of maternal and child health services and centers (which began between 1900 and 1910), better housing and sanitation, and higher levels of education accompanied by a general rise in living standards.

The most important factor has been improvement in infant and child feeding, associated with the introduction of safe milk, processed infant foods, mixtures based on cow's milk, and the education of mothers in hygienic feeding methods. Greater reliance on breast milk has played no part in reducing infant mortality in the affluent countries [italics added], though it was strongly advocated by Newman and other authorities. In fact breast feeding has declined almost to the vanishing point during the last 40 to 50 years in most of these countries, a period that has seen a transformation in infant and child health.

Experience thus suggests that PCM (protein-calorie malnutrition) can be eliminated in a few decades by the establishment of adequate maternal and child health services, rising standards of living, and hygienic artificial feeding. Examples of this can be found not only in highly developed countries in the temperate zone, but also in poor countries in the tropics, e.g., Barbados and Puerto Rico. In unusual circumstances, the change can actually take place "at one bound," so to speak. With M. A. Hossain (2), the author showed that when a community from an underdeveloped country was transferred to a well-developed country and adopted the infant feeding practices of the latter, its infant mortality rate immediately fell to something near the level prevailing in the new country. In this instance the fall took place in a Pakistani community that migrated to Bradford in Yorkshire, and affected the first infants born to women who had left home to join their husbands. The infantile mortality rate in the part of Pakistan from which the families came was about 150. In Bradford it was 45. The new environment meant, among other things, an abundance of cheap cow's milk in various forms and an absence of serious intestinal infections. Perhaps the most remarkable thing was the immediate and almost complete abandonment of breast feeding by the immigrant mothers, in spite of the fact that in Pakistan breast feeding is the accepted and traditional infant feeding practice, and an infant who is not breast-fed has little chance of survival.

After further consideration of the alternatives of breast feeding and artificial feeding, Aykroyd concludes:

Given these facts, the best approach to the problem of PCM seems at first sight to be to encourage breast feeding, to promote its retention where it still persists, or to promote a return to the practice where it has been abandoned. This is in line with the teaching of many authorities. But hitherto all attempts to do this have failed everywhere in the world, for reasons that have not been adequately studied. There do not seem to be any real prospects of retaining breast feeding in the spreading urban areas in the tropics where malnutrition is common and serious. Further, in the affluent countries, the virtual disappearance of breast feeding, the general use of processed cow's milk in the feeding of infants and young children, and the elimination of protein-calorie malnutrition have all coincided.

A more promising method of preventing PCM in the developing countries is to encourage the production and use of cheap feeding mixtures, based largely on plant foods that can fulfill the needs of the growing infant. A small percentage of milk powder enhances the nutritive value of such mixtures. Maternal and child health services and centers would, of course, be needed to teach mothers how to handle these mixtures and how to avoid infection. In other words, the aim would be a satisfactory artificial infant food made without cow's milk or with very little of it. The general adoption of this method of infant feeding in developing countries would not prevent the use of processed cow's milk preparations by those who could afford them nor breast feeding by mothers who favored it.

Aykroyd (1) reiterates in his summary:

Experience in the affluent countries has shown that this complex can be rapidly eliminated by efficient health services, rising standards of living, and hygienic artificial feeding. Greater reliance on breast feeding has played no part in its disappearance. The most promising method of attacking PCM in the developing countries is to promote the production and use of cheap feeding mixtures, based on plant foods that fulfill the infant's needs for calories, protein, and other nutrients.

I have quoted this at length because of the apparent lack of perspective manifest by some today who have not troubled to examine how the present state of infant care in our industrialized society has evolved.

"THEN THE WHINING SCHOOL-GIRL"

The velocity of growth of the child decreases from birth to 6–8 years, and nutritional demands are less in proportion to energy needs. The school girl, however, experiences a prepubertal spurt of growth at about 9 or 10 years of age, some 2 years earlier than that of boys. Indeed, she may become taller and larger at that period than a boy of the same age. At this time her energy requirement increases. As growth slows and puberty is followed by menstruation, nutrient demands undergo further alteration.

During subsequent adolescent growth, the energy requirement reaches a plateau, but requirements for protein, calcium, and other essential nutrients increase (11, 13). Hence, there is a greater need for food of high nutrient density. With the onset of menstruation, iron loss markedly increases, and the dietary allowance of this nutrient very nearly doubles, from 10 mg/day to 18 mg/day. It remains at this high level throughout the child-bearing ages—"the lover sighing like a furnace."

"AND THEN THE WIFE"

Woman's requirement of iron as a result of her physiologic loss is in decided contrast to man's need. Her requirement may become greatly exaggerated due to abnormal menstrual losses, common among women until completion of the menopause. These facts account for the prevalence of iron deficiency anemia among women in contrast to its relatively infrequent occurrence in men.

It behooves us to consider a widely misunderstood consequence of this physiologic need of iron by women (3). Diets in the United States, Sweden, and similar, industrially developed countries supply less than 6 mg iron/1000 kcal, or about 10–12 mg iron, daily for a woman who consumes 2000 calories. The recommended dietary allowance of iron for a woman during the reproductive period is 18 mg/day. This amount cannot be supplied by her diet, which is limited to an intake of some 2000 calories, without the addition or restoration of iron to the food supply. It is not possible for a large proportion of the population with a critical need for iron, i.e., women during the reproductive period, to have an adequate intake of iron as recommended by authorities without enhancing the iron content of our food supply. In the developing countries, the diet contains much larger quantities of iron than in developed countries, as a result of less care in the handling of raw foodstuffs and the opportunity for iron-containing contamination. The major difference is the less rigorous standards exercised for cleaning and storing of raw cereals and the resulting premilling exposure to contamination. This point is obvious from the geographically broad studies made by the Interdepartmental Committee on Nutrition for National Defense (Development), which revealed that the average iron content of diets in country after country—ranging from the lowest in the Philippines (14–39.6 mg daily) to the highest in Ethiopia (98–1418 mg daily)— all well above the levels in the United States. The recommendations relative to increasing the iron content of cereal foodstuffs made by the Food and Drug Administration are well conceived and sound. They should be supported as a means of bringing the American dietary intake of iron to the level that will safely meet the normal needs of women.

"AND THEN THE WIFE, HER FAIR ROUND BELLY
WITH GROWING FETUS LIN'D"

The nutritional demands of the reproductive interlude—pregnancy and lactation—are dealt with in the chapters by Thomson, McGanity, Delgado, and Filer. The added needs of women during pregnancy and lactation vary from culture to culture, depending upon their size; the level of physical activity maintained; the length of lactation; reserves of nutrients with which they enter pregnancy; concomitant demands of chronic disease states resulting from parasitic infestations such as hookworm or schistosomisis; and a variety of other sociocultural, environmental, and economically related factors (10).

The magnitude of these needs has been estimated from a variety of studies. The methodologies include direct determination of the composition of fetuses and stillborn infants and placental tissues, the composition and quantitative production of milk, indirect measures of maternal and infant composition, chemical determination of losses and patterns of change in the nutrient levels of body fluids during pregnancy and lactation, as well as direct observation of dietary intakes. Resultant allowances, such as those of the Recommended Dietary Allowances (RDA) (13) or the WHO/FAO Recommended Intake of Nutrients (11), provide reasoned guidelines to the desirable increments in nutrient intakes during pregnancy and lactation consistent with maintaining a state judged clinically to be healthy.

The RDAs provide (13) for caloric increments of 300 and 500 kcal and increases of 30 and 20 g protein daily, respectively, for pregnancy and lactation. Percentage increments of other nutrients, range from 20–50% for vitamin A, 50% for calcium, and 50–100% for folacin. The increments in most other vitamins and minerals are in the range of 25–40% above those allowances for nonpregnant women. Vitamin D, for which there is no RDA for adults, is needed during pregnancy and lactation in amounts comparable to the recommended intake of growing children. Iron constitutes a special case, in that supplements of 30–60 mg are recommended during pregnancy, an amount that cannot be obtained from the diet in the United States.

Since the recommended increment of energy intake is but some 15%, it is apparent that the diet of the pregnant woman must be carefully planned to provide more foods of higher nutrient density than are required during the nonpregnant state. A corollary is that less of those foods of low nutrient density may be included in her daily fare.

Some aspects of new experimental findings concerning trace elements (12) may have future implications in practice. Worthy of note are the potential implications of recent investigations concerning trace elements and the dependence of the animal organism upon a continuous, almost daily, extrinsic supply to meet high demands of certain localized tissue processes. Interference with such processes may result from a brief period of dietary restriction, lasting only 3–5 days, despite a previously abundant intake of zinc and the absence of measurable changes in the body stores of this element. It appears that mobilization of zinc from body stores is possible, but the rate of mobilization is not sufficiently labile for the intrinsic stores to meet the greatly enhanced localized requirements that may occur as a result of rapid tissue synthesis in processes such as wound healing or crucial periods of rapid fetal development. Studies of this phenomenon during gestation are limited to the lower species at present, but these findings highlight a need to investigate the effect of the relatively short periods of restricted nutrient intake frequently experienced by women early in pregnancy. Investigations of this and the possible roles of other trace elements in the development of the human fetus undoubtedly will receive much attention in the years ahead.

"THE LEAN AND SLIPPERED PANTALOON"

The special requirements of the reproductive-aged woman disappear (11, 13) as she reaches the age of "the lean and slippered pantaloon," as her requirements are no longer conditioned by reproduction and her menstrual losses. By this age, her basal metabolic rate has gradually lowered, and her activity often decreases. The "T.V. on the side" is in part responsible for the latter, especially if she is partially incapacitated by any disability or has limited social contacts. Recommended energy allowances are decreased by some 15% in recognition of these changes with age, but there is *no* significant decrease in the estimated allowances of other nutrients except iron. Accordingly, once more, she has need to include generous proportions of foods of high nutrient density in order to maintain good nutriture.

Other factors may be the older woman's motivation to prepare food and to eat. Without detailing the variants, it is evident that psychologic states of loneliness, dependency, absence of social anticipation, relative immobility, to say nothing of financial limitations, may deter her from partaking of a nutritionally healthy diet—and thus contribute, if not to her exit from the stage, at least to the loss of comfort and well-being as she moves behind the curtain.

This volume brings together aspects of nutrition relative to the health of women which previously have not been assembled in one place. In so doing, it will broaden the understanding of nutritionists and dietitians, gynecologists, obstetricians, pediatricians, and internists about their responsibilities for guiding the nutritionally more vulnerable sex throughout life. Investigators from these many fields of human biology will find in the following chapters challenges to undertake fruitful and important research.

REFERENCES

1. Aykroyd WR: Nutrition and mortality in infancy and early childhood: past and present relationships. Am J Clin Nutr 24:480, 1971
2. Aykroyd WR, Hossain MA: Diet and state of nutrition of Pakistani infants in Bradford, Yorkshire. Br Med J 1:42, 1967

3. Darby WJ: The case for the proposed increase in iron enrichment of flour and wheat products. Nutr Rev 30:98, 1972
4. Fomon SJ: Infant Nutrition. Philadelphia, WB Saunders, 1967
5. Halas ES, Hanlon MJ, Sandstead HH: Intra-uterine nutrition and aggression. Nature 257:221, 1975
6. Hytten FE, Leitch J: The Physiology of Human Pregnancy. Oxford, Blackwell, 1964
7. Maternal Nutrition and the Course of Pregnancy. Washington DC, Committee on Maternal Nutrition, Food and Nutrition Board, National Research Council, National Academy of Sciences, 1970
8. McKenzie JM, Fosmire GJ, Sandstead HH: Zinc deficiency during the latter third of pregnancy: effects on fetal rat brain, liver, and placenta. J Nutr 105:1466, 1975
9. Newman G: Infant Mortality, a Social Problem. London, Methuen, 1906
10. Nutrition in Pregnancy and Lactation. (Tech Rep No. 302). Geneva, 1965
11. Passmore R, Nicol BM, Narayana Rao M: Handbook on Human Nutritional Requirements. (Monograph No. 61). Geneva, WHO, 1974
12. Prasad A (ed): Trace elements and human disease, 2 vols. A Nutrition Foundation Monograph, New York, Academic Press (In press)
13. Recommended Dietary Allowances. Committee on Dietary Allowances, Food and Nutrition Board, National Research Council. Washington DC, National Academy of Sciences, 1974
14. Simon (Sir) J: Cited by Aykroyd, 1861
15. Toverud KU, Stearns G, Macy IG: Maternal nutrition and child health, an interpretive review. Bulletin of the National Research Council No. 123. Washington DC, National Academy of Sciences-National Research Council, 1950

Chapter 2

Physiologic Basis of Nutritional Needs During Pregnancy and Lactation

Angus M. Thomson, Frank E. Hytten

Physiologists and biochemists have studied the metabolism of pregnant women for more than a century. But since it is far from easy to make accurate physiologic observations on healthy pregnant and lactating women, knowledge of metabolic and functional changes during human reproduction has progressed very slowly and erratically from a fragmented to a reasonably organized state. The subject is still not being taught in many medical schools, and it has not yet been incorporated into many standard textbooks of human physiology. Probably the first comprehensive attempt to review the literature from the point of view of human nutrition was Hytten and Leitch's monograph *The Physiology of Human Pregnancy*, first published in 1964, with a greatly expanded second edition in 1971 (18).

Obstetricians—being busy, practical people—could not afford to wait for accurate physiologic information before giving nutritional advice to their patients. Somewhat surprisingly, their advice has often been restrictive. Around the turn of the century, Prochownick (32) claimed that restricting intakes of food and fluids helped to reduce the risk of difficult labor. A few decades later, many obstetricians, especially those in the United States, were insisting that pregnant women should eat less and gain less weight in order to prevent pregnancy toxemia (8). At the same time, supplements of vitamins and minerals were prescribed freely.

Nutritionists considered that pregnant and lactating women formed vulnerable groups exposed to special dangers of malnutrition because of their increased dietary requirements. Hence, nutritional generosity should be beneficial from the point of view of public health and personal welfare. This view was strongly supported by the fact that the successful food rationing policy in Great Britain during World War II was accompanied by a remarkable fall in perinatal mortality rates that could not easily be explained *except* in terms of better maternal nutrition (9). Burke and her colleagues reported a close correlation between the nutritive value of the diets of pregnant women in Boston, Massachusetts, and the condition of their babies (1).

Yet paradoxes and difficulties accumulated which stimulated renewed interest in the metabolic nature of human reproduction. Burke's findings were not supported by subsequent surveys (27, 39). A severe famine in Holland during 1944–1945 caused a small reduction in birth weights, with only minor adverse effect on perinatal mortality rates (37). Populations are increasing rapidly, and breast-feeding is widespread in countries with chronically poor nutritional conditions. It appears as if human reproduction is not quite so vulnerable to nutritional adversity as we used to think.

To reconcile and understand such puzzling phenomena, it is essential to know more about the physiologic basis of human reproduction. In this short review, we will discuss some of the philosophic and practical problems with which we have been concerned, using factual illustrations as necessary.

THE ORGANIZATION OF PHYSIOLOGIC RESEARCH ON PREGNANT AND LACTATING WOMEN

In general medicine and surgery, research on metabolism and other physiologic functions is undertaken mostly on sick patients, who are physically confined to a hospital bed and psychologically receptive to investigation. It is otherwise with healthy pregnant or lactating women, who go about their normal business except for a short period during and after delivery and periodically attend out-patient clinics for the purposes of medical supervision. Much of the earlier physiologic research was undertaken on women admitted to the hospital because of abnormalities; these women could scarcely be regarded as normal and physiologic.

Research on the physiology of human pregnancy necessitates the provision of special facilities which are attractive to healthy women. Even then, selection is necessary. The physiologic responses of a bright-eyed young primigravida from a good home may not be the same as those of a woman living in poverty who has borne several children in quick succession. It is desirable to choose women who are not only physically healthy but also intelligent and likely to cooperate reliably, if necessary over a considerable period of time. Without careful selection on such lines, losses through inadequate cooperation may be heavy. Women who volunteer for research which may not benefit them personally deserve and respond to administrative and medical arrangements which ensure that they receive clinical care of a high technical order under conditions which cater to their human as well as medical needs. This implies continuity of personnel, an effective appointments system, comfortable physical surroundings, assistance with transport if desired, and so on. To all these must be added scientific resources which ensure that measurements and observations are as accurate as possible.

Given good scientific and clinical conditions, together with cooperative patients, our experience is that healthy women will submit readily to procedures which may be painful, time-consuming, occasionally undignified, and even dangerous. We, therefore, have a rigorous procedure for ethical supervision of research and for obtaining informed consent from patients. Projects, after being discussed with clinically experienced senior colleagues who are not involved in the research, are submitted formally to an official Ethics Committee which includes lay (including legal) representatives as well as medical and scientific representatives. Written permission to proceed must be obtained from the Committee, and its members have an absolute right to veto any proposal. Finally, in the presence of a witness, a research worker explains the project to each individual patient, who is told that if she prefers not to cooperate, the clinical care she receives will not be prejudiced. We do not ask patients to sign a consent form. Instead, the responsible doctor and the witness note on the record that the procedure has been explained and that the patient has freely agreed to volunteer.

In addition to this, one must have the necessary technical resources. The clinical accommodation of our Unit includes sanitary facilities, and also a small kitchen. The laboratories are adjacent so that specimens can be handed over and dealt with quickly and conveniently. These resources are backed by those of a hospital, and a university, from which the advice and help of specialists can be obtained when desired. The research unit itself is multidisciplinary, the scientific staff including obstetricians, physiologists, a biochemist, and a statistician.

EMPIRICAL EVIDENCE

A first approximation to defining nutritional needs can be obtained by surveying reproductive behavior. If a woman remains healthy during pregnancy, produces a living baby of high vitality, is capable of satisfactory lactation, and recovers smoothly, then her diet is, by definition, likely to be nutritionally satisfactory; furthermore, the level where nutritional inadequacy begins may theoretically be defined by looking for associations between limited supplies of nutrients and abnormal clinical phenomena.

We began our investigations 25 years ago by making dietary and clinical surveys in Aberdeen, Scotland. A group of primigravidas was asked to cooperate in 1-week weighed dietary surveys during the seventh month of pregnancy, that time being chosen because the fetus would be growing rapidly, most women had given up paid work, and few abnormalities of late pregnancy had appeared. In addition to measuring and analyzing food intakes as carefully as possible, accurate clinical records of pregnancy, labor and the puerperium, including measurements of weight change, were kept. When the records were complete, we compared dietary and clinical data in the hope of defining a point at which decreasing intake of nutrients was associated with an increasing incidence of abnormalities. We were not successful, although many of the women apparently took diets with an energy and nutrient intake well below the recommended dietary allowances (39). The Vanderbilt team, which made a similar survey in Tennessee, also obtained predominantly negative results (27). We were forced to conclude that, under conditions in Britain and the United States during the 1950s, a remarkably wide range of dietary intakes during pregnancy was compatible with a satisfactory clinical outcome.

Our data also showed that tall primigravidas had much more satisfactory clinical histories than did short primigravidas (40). If tallness can be interpreted as indicating satisfactory previous growth, the lifetime nutritional experience of the mother might be as important as what she ate after she became pregnant.

These findings appeared at a time when most nutritionists believed that the diets of pregnant women were of critical importance, and they were received with skepticism. Yet, they have stood the test of time. We know of only one satisfactory field demonstration that improving the food supply, especially in terms of energy, improves reproductive efficiency. This was made in an impoverished rural community in Guatemala by Lechtig et al. (23). Again, there has been widespread confirmation of our finding that maternal physique has an important influence on reproductive performance.

We concluded in 1959 (39) that

the diets of pregnant women can vary widely, in quantity as well as in quality, without clinically obvious impairment of the reproductive process. But although the importance of diet in pregnancy is usually inconspicuous in terms of the individual mother and child, the same is not necessarily true in terms of large populations.

Those conclusions are still valid. The problem is to explain, in physiologic terms, why that is so.

FETAL PRIORITIES AND MATERNAL ADAPTATIONS

The simplest concept of gestation is to assume that the mother and the product of conception, the fetus, are physiologically independent organisms separated by a filter, the placenta, through which the fetus acquires the nutrients it needs. The question is: What happens if the food intake of the mother is insufficient for the sum of maternal and fetal needs? Does the fetus behave as a parasite, taking what it needs by depleting the maternal tissues, if necessary, or is the mother able to conserve her own resources by limiting supplies to the fetus? In accordance with the empirical evidence already summarized, it appears that the fetus, though by no means a perfect parasite, is remarkably efficient at obtaining what it needs even when the maternal diet is not abundant. This makes evolutionary sense because, if it were not so, the mammalian reproductive process might not suffice to ensure the survival of the species.

The earliest physiologic evidence, taken from feeding experiments on animals, was interpreted as signifying that "the maternal tissues are taking precedence over the nutrition of the fetus" (31). This view was reversed by the results of human balance experiments; for example, nitrogen balances in relatively well-nourished women indicated that far more nitrogen was being stored during pregnancy than could be accounted for in the reproductive organs and the product of conception (25). In 1919, Slemons (36) concluded that normal pregnancy "represents for the mother a gain rather than a sacrifice and accordingly her tissues are not deprived of material to supply the new organism." Only if the maternal diet became seriously inadequate would the fetus tend to grow at the expense of maternal tissues. We now know that the classic balance experiments indicated retentions which were far too high, no doubt because intakes were overestimated and outputs underestimated; more recent nitrogen balance studies show retentions of a much more modest order (22, 46). The earlier data, combined with enthusiasm for providing synthetic vitamins and concentrates of nutrients to pregnant and lactating women, undoubtedly caused nutrient requirements during pregnancy and lactation to be overestimated. In 1946, Garry and Wood (11) emphasized the lack of reliable physiologic evidence and suggested that the absence of clinical confirmation was leading to "the development of a more critical attitude, even of disillusionment."

When evidence is scanty, we are obliged to speculate. Hammond, in 1944 (14), suggested that nutrients in the maternal blood stream are partitioned in accordance with the metabolic rate of tissues, the product of conception coming second only to the maternal central nervous system. This theory still lives; Hammond's diagram was reproduced in 1975 by Schneider and Dancis (35) with the comment that "Consistent with its rapid growth rate, it [the fetus] receives more nutrition per unit weight than does the mother." The theory rests on the proposition that fetal energy metabolism per unit weight is considerably above that of the mother. True, the fetus is growing rapidly, but it does not have to maintain body heat against an adverse temperature gradient, and it has a relatively low muscle tone before delivery. Hytten and Leitch (18) calculated from published measurements that the total energy needs of the uterus and its contents are "a little higher than when the total is taken in proportion to maternal basal metabolism, but in sensible agreement with it." If so, it is necessary to conclude that the fetus does not depend for its efficiency on a relatively high rate of energy metabolism.

Energy, however, is by no means the whole story. Levels of many (but not all) nutrients in the blood of pregnant women are lower than those found in nonpregnant women (19); conversely, levels in the fetal circulation are often higher than those in the maternal (4). It has often been assumed that such phenomena represent deprivation of maternal tissues by the fetus acting as an extremely competent parasite. The idea is plausible and has great practical significance; enormous quantities of vitamins and minerals are prescribed to protect mothers against hypothetical deprivation. Yet the theory that the fetus causes mothers to teeter on the verge of deficiency is shaky, to say the least.

If falling levels of nutrients in maternal blood are due to the fetus' depleting maternal reserves, one would expect no such effect to occur during the first half of pregnancy, at the end of which the fetus plus placenta weighs less than 500 g. But most of the putative signs of maternal deprivation are established well before that time. For example, the maternal serum albumin level falls during the first trimester, when the gain of protein by the product of conception is trivial. Whatever causes the fall in maternal levels, it can scarcely be fetal requirements.

Even if that were possible, the evidence is equivocal. Maternal hemoglobin concentrations do fall during pregnancy, a fact usually interpreted as showing that fetal demands for iron, which increase considerably during the final trimester, are depleting maternal iron reserves. Yet there is abundant evidence that the total amount of hemoglobin in the maternal circulation *increases* during pregnancy, even when extra iron is not provided (30). Furthermore, it has been established by using isotopes that pregnant women are able to increase the percentage of dietary iron absorbed (15). The fall in hemoglobin concentration per unit volume of blood is due to a relatively greater increase in plasma volume. A possible reason for the latter is the need to increase heat flow through the maternal skin and to expand renal plasma flow.

In our experience, the subject of "anemia" has a highly emotive content, even to the extent that physicians who fail to give iron pills to healthy pregnant women may be considered negligent. Without going so far, it is commonly argued that giving additional iron is at best beneficial and at worst harmless. The situation may not be quite so simple, and in our view, the subject is fit for further research—not therapeutic dogmatism.

We know that concentrations of most nutrients and metabolites in maternal blood fall during pregnancy—for example, nearly all electrolytes; total protein, albumin and probably γ-globulin, urea, creatinine, glucose, and some amino acids; folate, vitamin B_{12}, ascorbic acid, and pyridoxine. On the other hand, some levels rise—for example, α- and β-globulins and some amino acids; total lipids, triglycerides, cholesterol, phospholipids, and free fatty acids. These changes are accompanied by many other biophysical and biochemical alterations in the properties of maternal blood: for example, reduced osmolality, accelerated erythrocyte sedimentation rates, and changed enzyme levels. It is worth emphasizing that such changes are to be found in perfectly healthy pregnant women and that most can be discerned in early pregnancy. They must, therefore, represent processes of physiologic adaptation rather than nutritional depletion or excess. Unless this is understood, nutritional illness may be diagnosed where none exists, and treatment given which is unnecessary or potentially harmful (19).

However, there are some aspects of physiologic adaptation during pregnancy which must be regarded as potentially harmful until proved otherwise. For example, alterations in kidney function result in considerable losses of some nutrients (for example, many amino acids) in urine (17). It appears that glycosuria, which undoubtedly becomes more common during pregnancy, may be caused by altered renal function rather than by the altered carbohydrate metabolism which is also present (5).

Such phenomena require much more investigation. All that can be said at present is that the boundary between physiology and pathology becomes blurred during pregnancy; pathology should be diagnosed by reference to gestation-specific standards of normality derived from healthy pregnant women and not to standards which have been derived from nonpregnant individuals. Well-intentioned nutritional prophylactic regimens should be used with a skeptical frame of mind and with caution. As Leitch (24) pointed out nearly 20 years ago, Claude Bernard's famous dictum about the importance of a constant *milieu intérieur* has to be modified in its application to pregnancy.

The metabolic adaptations of pregnancy are no doubt induced by the temporary endocrinologic changes which have long been recognized as essential to the pregnant state. From the standpoint of endocrinology, the mother and the fetus cannot be regarded as two physiologically independent organisms. Rather, the mother and the product of conception form a symbiotic whole, acting and reacting upon each other. We can at present only speculate about the reasons behind the altered metabolic conditions of pregnancy. Hytten and Leitch (18) sum up as follows:

It is reasonable to assume that, in health, the body maintains in its fluid environment the amounts and concentrations of the substance it needs for maximum efficiency of function; that is the purpose of homeostasis. If that is so then the greatly altered amounts and concentrations which are characteristic of pregnancy cannot reasonably be assumed to be equally advantageous to the mother's metabolism. The most plausible explanation is that they represent changes which allow maximum efficiency of fetal growth and metabolism. The fetus, using hormones as manipulators, overrides and resets the mother's homeostatic mechanisms in its own interests; it is the price of viviparity.

We see no reason to alter that general concept. However, well-intentioned attempts to restore maternal biochemistry to nonpregnant levels by means of nutritional and therapeutic interventions may not be entirely harmless to the fetus. In our view, maternal adaptations during pregnancy should be regarded as potentially beneficial to the fetus unless there is clear proof that they are harmful.

Much less is known of lactation. There is no reason to suppose that it is accompanied by large-scale metabolic adjustments in the maternal organism. Here, mother and baby are physiologically independent individuals, changes in the mother being restricted to the regression of her metabolism to a nonpregnant condition on which only those modifications which are necessary for the secretion of milk are superimposed. Maternal fertility is, however, modified to some extent by breast-feeding, a possible mechanism being that suckling stimulates a hypothalamic response that stimulates the pituitary to produce prolactin and at the same time inhibits gonadotrophin production (3). However, even the elementary facts are not yet adequately established; for example, vast differences in the timing of the return of menstruation after parturition have been reported (44).

The only other specific question we shall refer to is that of the efficiency, in terms of energy, of human milk production. The situation in human females is not analogous to that of animals, which may have to produce enough milk for large litters or have been conditioned by selective breeding to produce far more milk than is required for the nutrition of their young. In cattle, the availability of metabolizable energy for the secretion of milk appears to be about 69% (33). In women, FAO (10) estimated the conversion efficiency to be 60%. On that basis, the provision of human milk with an energy value of 600 kcal would involve the mother's consuming 1000 kcal of metabolizable energy in addition to her ordinary needs, i.e., up to 50% more than the intake of an average nonpregnant, nonlactating woman. Since successfully lactating women do not have such conspicuously large appetites, this estimate seemed to us implausible. We calculated from our own data that the efficiency of human milk production is probably around 90% (43). In general, it appears that milk production by women is possible at a cost which is scarcely more than the nutritive value of the milk itself. Since women living under poor nutritional conditions are surprisingly successful, it appears that mothers have a considerable ability to subsidize lactation from their own tissues. The evolutionary value of such efficiency is obvious.

THE ROLE OF THE PLACENTA

It has been known for many years that average weights of fetuses and newborn babies, plotted against gestational age, form an S-shaped curve, the apparent rate of growth falling off during the final weeks of gestation. This has usually been interpreted as a result of terminal "placental insufficiency." The concept is that unless the fetus is exposed to some form of nutritional restriction, its growth curve would be nearly linear from an early stage of pregnancy until parturition, and that the limits of the ability of the placenta to transfer nutrients are frequently reached before the end of normal pregnancy. The idea seems reasonable, but little or no direct evidence in support has become available; in a recent treatise there seems to be general agreement that the role of the placenta itself in limiting supplies is small compared to that of the supply line to the placenta (13). In other words, placental insufficiency probably has no basis in physiologic fact and is not even commonly the result of placental pathology; bottlenecks in the supply line to the fetus should be looked for in the maternal blood supply to the placenta. It is tempting to adopt the stance that, for example, small women have more restricted circulations than tall women, and that is why they have smaller babies with higher mortality rates. Yet the demonstration that the "litter weight" in twin pregnancies is far higher than that of singleton babies and shows little sign of growth retardation before term (6, 28) makes us hesitate to accept any simple mechanistic hypothesis. Hill (16) has shown that removing one lobe of the bidiscoid placentas of rhesus monkeys causes a considerable degree of fetal growth retardation, but the moral may be more relevant to the pathology than to the physiology of human gestation. Available facts suggest that the human placenta has a large functional reserve, even near term.

There have been few claims that the composition of maternal blood is directly correlated with the growth rate and composition of the fetus (2, 21). It should be noted that the physiologic role of the placenta is by no means that of a passive filter of nutrients and fetal waste products. Gases—and possibly some simple solutes—may indeed pass freely through the endotheliotrophoblastic barrier. But for more complex molecules, there are processes of facilitated or active transfer. We have already referred to the fact that many substances exist in higher concentration in the fetal than the maternal blood, which suggests a "one-way traffic" in favor of the fetus. A probable explanation is that some nutrients are converted during their passage through the placenta or during circulation in the fetus into biochemical forms which cannot pass so freely in the reverse direction (4). For example, ascorbic acid passes through placenta as dehydroascorbic acid and is converted on the fetal side to L-ascorbic acid, to which the placenta is much less permeable.

Such fragments of evidence suggest that the placenta, in addition to being highly efficient, also plays an active role favoring the nutrition of the fetus and functions as a fetal excretory organ and a ductless gland. Further progress in understanding placental function may not be easy until we obtain a satisfactory model whereby functions can be studied *in vitro* using living human placental tissue. Indirect methods of study in the intact organism appear to be near the limits of present technology; and it seems unlikely that much further understanding can be achieved through anatomic and pathologic examinations.

NUTRITIONAL IMPLICATIONS OF CHANGES IN BODY COMPOSITION

The determination of changes in body composition, one might call it "biochemical dissection," has proved to be a very useful approach to the problem of estimating nutritional needs during pregnancy (18).

Our starting point was that the average weight gain of healthy pregnant women eating to appetite averaged 12.5 kg (41), of which only about 8 kg could be accounted for by known components: the fetus, placenta, amniotic fluid, growth of the uterus and mammary glands, and increase of maternal blood volume. What was the rest?

When we started to consider this problem, there were two strong candidates: protein and water. Protein can only be stored as cytoplasm containing at least 80% water, and on this basis we expected to find that the missing 4.5 kg would be accounted for by at least 4 liters of gained water. We were prepared to disregard the large amounts of stored protein that had been indicated by balance experiments on the grounds that the apparent retentions of nitrogen had been overestimated; if large retentions of protein had indeed occurred, adding the necessary amount of associated water resulted in estimates of weight to be gained which were far in excess of those observed.

We measured gains in total body water during pregnancy using deuterium oxide as the tracer (20). Unexpectedly, women with no more than minimal edema proved to have only about 1½ liters of extra water at term, in addition to that which could be accounted for in the product of conception, the organs of reproduction, and the increased maternal blood volume. On the assumption that most of this small excess of water was extracellular, we were forced to conclude that any "surplus" protein stored by the mother was trivial or nonexistent. The 4.5-kg weight to be accounted for therefore could not be protein, nor was it likely to be carbohydrate. Only about one-third of the weight was water. The rest, about 3 kg, must be fat. The fat storage hypothesis—that of a large increase in depot fat—received direct semi-quantitative support from serial skinfold measurements in pregnant women who were eating to appetite (38).

There was, however, a curious anomaly: many of the carefully selected healthy pregnant women we studied had exhibited signs of generalized edema and had stored such considerable amounts of water (even when the extent of edema was clinically inconspicuous) that we had to assume that they had gained much less fat than women who had not exhibited generalized edema. Since every medical student is taught that edema is pathologic, we were thus faced with the unlikely situation that some 40% of carefully chosen women who had had perfectly normal pregnancies in all other respects were apparently "pathologic." The hospital kept unusually good clinical records, and we were able to show that some 40% of all nonhypertensive pregnant women were indeed recorded as exhibiting some degree of edema (42), so our own sample seemed to be typical enough. A further intensive study showed that edema can be found in the great majority of healthy pregnant women if looked for carefully (34). Where, then, is the water stored? We have not attempted to answer this question experimentally, but there are strong indications in the literature that large amounts of free water can be stored in the mucopolysaccharides of connective tissue (12). This seems to make sense physiologically, since it is well known that connective tissue in pregnant women becomes much more stretchable, for example, in the symphysis pubis and the areolae of the nipples. Clearly, there is still a great deal to be learned about water metabolism during pregnancy.

An interesting feature of the skinfold measurements (38) was that they indicated extensive fat storage during the middle months of gestation, with little or no additional storage during the last trimester. The buffering effect of relatively early fat storage on the energy requirements of pregnancy is obvious. Instead of such requirements rising steeply at the end of pregnancy when the fetus is growing rapidly, they are spread over approximately 6 months. The maternal appetite increases sharply early in the second trimester and then levels off. Energy needs may be further buffered by diminished activity during late pregnancy. Anticipatory fat storage should assist fetal growth and survival if, perchance, the mother has to undergo nutritional deprivation at a later and more critical stage of pregnancy; it also provides a reserve of energy for lactation.

We were now able to account fairly accurately for the total amount of weight gained by pregnant women and to estimate the composition of its components. Calculations on this basis enabled us to make reasonable estimates of what might be termed the "capital gains" of various nutrients during pregnancy. To these must be added "running costs," for example, the raised basal metabolic rate of pregnancy. There may be other running costs. We have already referred to increased losses of some nutrients via the kidney. These may be compensated to some extent by increased efficiency in other respects, *e.g.*, improved absorption of nutrients through the intestine.

CONCLUSION

The present situation seems to be that we can specify, with reasonable accuracy, a nutritional strategy that should satisfy the nutritional needs of pregnant and lactating women who are physiologically normal, *i.e.*, women who are basically healthy and who are not exposed to unusual environmental stresses. These needs are less exacting than we thought 20 or 30 years ago, when the officially recommended additional allowances for pregnancy and lactation were considerably higher than they are now (7, 29, 45). Generous "guesstimates" have been replaced by lower estimates based on physiologic measurements, and excessively high measurements due to faulty techniques or erroneous assumptions have been supplanted by more reliable evidence. Healthy pregnant and lactating women quite rightly continue to be regarded as deserving special care, but we can now afford to discard the idea that they are hovering on the brink of undernutrition and malnutrition, even in communities that are generally well-fed.

This does not apply to communities where nutritional conditions are chronically and generally unsatisfactory. Even here, however, human reproduction is protected by powerful physiologic safeguards, and the improvements to be expected from dietary betterment are more likely to be discerned in statistical terms by means of such indices as perinatal mortality rates and mean birth weights than by reference to the clinical histories of individual women and small groups of women.

It is not sufficient to attend to nutrition during pregnancy and lactation only, because the anatomic and physiologic efficiency of women who have previously been exposed to malnutrition during the years of growth and development may be permanently impaired. McCarrison (26) summarized this concept nearly 40 years ago:

The satisfaction of nutritional needs in pregnancy begins with the antenatal lives of the mothers of our race. It must continue during the period of their growth up to, during and following the period when they find their fulfilment in motherhood; a fulfilment for which nutrition prepares and makes ready the way.

It is worth adding that malnutrition usually forms part of a generally unsatisfactory environment arising from poverty, lack of education, and limited material resources. Therefore, nutritional measures should form part of a wider spectrum of improvement.

Whatever the conditions, we need continuing research on the rather vague boundary between physiology and pathology; on the fact that pregnant women have unusual metabolic patterns which sometimes change abruptly from physiology to pathology; and on the mechanisms whereby the fetus is able to secure and to safeguard its own nutritional needs.

REFERENCES

1. Burke BS, Stuart HC: Nutritional requirements during pregnancy and lactation. JAMA 137: 119, 1948
2. Churchill JA, Moghissi KS, Evans TN, Frohman C: Relationships of maternal amino acid blood levels to fetal development. Obstet Gynecol 33:492, 1969
3. Coppola JA: Brain catecholamines and gonadotropin secretion. In Martini L. Ganong WF (eds): Frontiers in Neuroendocrinology. New York, Oxford University Press, 1971, p 129
4. Dancis J, Schneider H: Physiology: transfer and barrier function. In Gruenwald P (ed): The Placenta and its Maternal Supply Line. Lancaster, Engl, MTP, 1975, pp 98–124
5. Davison JM, Hytten FE: The effect of pregnancy on the renal handling of glucose. Br J Obstet Gynaecol 82:374, 1975

6. Daw E, Walker J: Biological aspects of twin pregnancy in Dundee. Br J Obstet Gynaecol 82:29, 1975
7. Department of Health and Social Security: Recommended intakes of nutrients for the United Kingdom. Report on Public Health and Medical Subjects No. 120, 1970
8. Dieckmann WJ: The Toxemias of Pregnancy, 2nd ed. London, Henry Kimpton, 1952
9. Duncan EHL, Baird D, Thomson AM: The causes and prevention of stillbirths and first week deaths. 1. The evidence of vital statistics. J Obstet Gynaecol Br Commonw 59:183, 1952
10. FAO: Calorie requirements. Rome, FAO Nutr Stud No. 15, 1957
11. Garry RC, Wood HO: Dietary requirements in human pregnancy and lactation. A review of recent work. Nutr Abstr Rev 15:591, 1946
12. Gersh I, Catchpole HR: The nature of ground substance of connective tissue. Perspect Biol Med 3:282, 1960
13. Gruenwald P: The supply line of the fetus; definitions relating to fetal growth. In Gruenwald P (ed): The Placenta and its Maternal Supply Line. Lancaster, Engl, MTP, 1975, pp 1–17
14. Hammond J: Physiological factors affecting birth weight. Proc Nutr Soc 2:8, 1944
15. Heinrich HC, Bartels H, Heinisch B, Hausmann K, Kuse R, Humke W, Mauss HJ: Intestinale ^{59}Fe-Resorption und prälatenter Eisenmangel während der Gravität des Menschen. Klin Wochenschr 46:199, 1968
16. Hill DE: Experimental growth retardation in rhesus monkeys. In Elliott K, Knight J (eds): Size at Birth. Amsterdam, Associated Scientific, 1974, p 99
17. Hytten FE, Cheyne GA: The aminoaciduria of pregnancy. J Obstet Gynaecol Br Commonw 79:424, 1972
18. Hytten FE, Leitch I: The Physiology of Human Pregnancy, 2nd ed. Oxford, Blackwell, 1971
19. Hytten FE, Lind T: Diagnostic Indices in Pregnancy. Basel, Ciba-Geigy, 1973
20. Hytten FE, Thomson AM, Taggart N: Total body water in normal pregnancy. J Obstet Gynaecol Br Commonw 73:553, 1966
21. Iyengar L, Rajalakshmi K: Effect of folic acid supplement on birth weights of infants. Am J Obstet Gynecol 122:332, 1975
22. Johnstone FD, MacGillivray I, Dennis KJ: Nitrogen retention in pregnancy. J Obstet Gynaecol Br Commonw 79:777, 1972
23. Lechtig A, Delgado H, Lasky R, Yarbrough C, Klein R, Habicht J–P, Behar M: Maternal nutrition and fetal growth in developing countries. Am J Dis Child 129:553, 1975
24. Leitch I: Changing concepts in the nutritional physiology of human pregnancy. Proc Nutr Soc 16:38, 1957
25. Macy IG, Hunscher HA: An evaluation of maternal nitrogen and mineral needs during embryonic and infant development. Am J Obstet Gynecol 27:878, 1934
26. McCarrison R: Nutritional needs in pregnancy. Br Med J 2:256, 1937
27. McGanity WJ, Cannon RO, Bridgforth EB, Martin MP, Densen PM, Newbill JA, McClellan GS, Christie A, Peterson JC, Darby WJ: The Vanderbilt cooperative study of maternal and infant nutrition VI. Relationship of obstetric performance to nutrition. Am J Obstet Gynecol 67:501, 1954
28. McKeown T, Record RG: Observations on foetal growth in multiple pregnancy in man. J Endocrinol 8:386, 1952
29. National Research Council: Recommended Dietary Allowances. Washington DC, National Academy of Sciences, 1974
30. Paintin DB, Thomson AM, Hytten FE: Iron and the haemoglobin level in pregnancy. J Obstet Gynaecol Br Commonw 73:181, 1966
31. Paton DN: The influence of diet in pregnancy on the weight of the offspring. Lancet 2:21, 1903
32. Prochownick L: An attempt towards the replacement of induced premature birth. Cbl Gynäk 13:577, 1889

33. Reid JT: Nutrition of lactating farm animals. In Kon SK, Cowie AT (eds): Milk: the Mammary Gland and its Secretion, Vol 2. New York, Academic Press, 1961, pp 47–87

34. Robertson EG: The natural history of oedema during pregnancy. J Obstet Gynaecol Br Commonw 78:520, 1971

35. Schneider H, Dancis J: Abnormalities of composition of maternal blood. In Gruenwald P (ed): The Placenta and its Maternal Supply Line. Lancaster, Engl MTP, 1975, pp 178–185

36. Slemons JM: The nutrition of the fetus. Am J Obstet Gynecol 80:194, 1919

37. Smith CA: The effect of wartime starvation in Holland upon pregnancy and its product. Am J Obstet Gynecol 53:599, 1947

38. Taggart NR, Holliday RM, Billewicz WZ, Hytten FE, Thomson AM: Changes in skinfolds during pregnancy. Br J Nutr 21:439, 1967

39. Thomson AM: Diet in pregnancy. 3. Diet in relation to the course and outcome of pregnancy. Br J Nutr 13: 509, 1959

40. Thomson AM: Maternal stature and reproductive efficiency. Eugenics Review 51:-155, 1959

41. Thomson AM, Billewicz WZ: Clinical significance of weight gains during pregnancy. Br Med J 1:243, 1957

42. Thomson AM, Hytten FE, Billewicz WZ: The epidemiology of oedema during pregnancy. J Obstet Gynaecol Br Commonw 74:1, 1967

43. Thomson AM, Hytten FE, Billewicz WZ: The energy cost of human lactation. Br J Nutr 24:565, 1970

44. Thomson AM, Hytten FE, Black AE: Lactation and reproduction. Bull WHO 52: 337, 1975.

45. WHO: Handbook on human nutritional requirements. (Monograph No. 61) Geneva, 1974

46. Zuspan FP, Goodrich S: Metabolic studies in normal pregnancy. 1. Nitrogen metabolism. Am J Obstet Gynecol 100:7, 1968

Chapter 3

The Implications of Undernutrition During Pubescence and Adolescence on Fertility

Samuel M. Wishik

The subject of this chapter is the confluence of factors that are covered in several chapters of this book, which face such questions as: 1) What effects do nutritional aberrations have on the favorable outcome of pregnancies among mature women? 2) What are the nutritional considerations during and around the time of adolescent change? and 3) What might preventive intervention contribute?

Within that framework, this chapter will focus on the interface between adolescent development and pregnancy potential and outcome, both as affected by undernutrition.

Avoiding the confusion that exists between physicians and demographers (and among the latter between those in France and in the United States) dictionaries define *fertility* as: producing offspring or the capacity to do so. We shall be referring to both—the capacity of the adolescent female to conceive and what happens if she does—both under the influence of undernutrition.

The different types of unfavorable outcome of pregnancy can be put on a continuum through time, ranging from failure to conceive to fetal failure (including faulty implantation, embryologic malformation, and interruption of pregnancy) to problems in childbirth to the liveborn child's experience as manifested in neonatal or postneonatal death and/or inadequacy of growth and development (22).

We shall concentrate on the first and the last—the first as exemplified in delayed menarche and anovulation, the last in the impaired growth and development of young children. But, in so doing, we recognize the statistical incompleteness of any universe under such research analysis and also the paradoxical effects that can follow attempts at promoting nutritional improvement. For example, a statistically unsignificant miscarriage might be moved up the continuum by improved nutrition to a more easily identifiable and measurable neonatal death.

On the subject of age of menarche, one is impressed particularly by the epidemiologic evidence, still with gaps and alternative interpretations, concerning secular change, population differences, and socioeconomic group membership. Therefore, certain assumptions will be made as if they were facts and discussed primarily with respect to possible influences concerning fertility. The assumptions are:

1. Undernutrition delays menarche (1, 8, 13).
2. Undernutrition delays the regularization of ovulation after menarche (1, 13, 20).
3. In other respects as well, undernutrition delays and interferes with post-menarcheal and postovulatory physiologic maturation and optimum readiness for reproduction.
4. Undernutrition modifies the pattern and timing of skeletal growth (2, 3, 20).

THE DELAY OF MENARCHE

Until recently, it was considered that the well-known spread of age of menarche is the type of genetically determined normal curve distribution that exists in most biologic phenomena and that this can be modified somewhat by nutrition. Frisch and her colleagues have further refined the nutritional component with her contention of the existence of a threshold of percent body fat (4, 5, 6, 9). She emphasizes the role of body fat stores, perhaps as energy sources for hormone production, although not in a direct sense, since the amount of energy involved immediately is minute. Of course, Frisch does not discount genetic influences, perhaps accepts those as contributing to pattern and rate of body development, including distribution among muscle, fat, and other tissues and water, and the complex factors affecting the competition between height and weight for available calories.

It seems, however, more reasonable to postulate a complementary balance between the force of the physiologic "drive" toward maturation and the availability of body mass or supportive fat stores, whatever the exact role played by the fat. We are searching to demonstrate a staircase-shaped threshold as the balance of drives shifts from fat storage to fat mobilization and utilization. Surely, the 7-year old is not likely to menstruate, regardless of her percent body fat score. Similarly, the 16-year old should be able to achieve menarche with a lower proportionate fat tissue reserve than the 12-year old. Frisch modifies her threshold level when applied to amenorrhea among adult women. This is consonant with the known capacity of grossly undernourished women in developing countries to remain fertile (19).

Our studies thus far, however, correlate well with Frisch's findings. Data on 608 school girls between 8 and 15 years of age in New Jersey, collected by Liskin, showed only 4 of 197 girls who fell below the Frisch threshold at menarche (11). In the same age-span, there were 85 nonmenstruating girls who were below the percent body fat threshold. Careful study of the data thus far failed to locate demarcation differences within the age-span. In any event, the significance of Frisch's work would not be lessened, in that the tremendous importance of attacking undernutrition as an essential part of the management of certain adolescent hypohormonal syndromes is highlighted.

DELAY IN REGULAR OVULATION

The relevance of age of menarche to fertility rests in the cyclic ovulation that is presaged by menarche. There is good reason to believe that earlier menarche advances the next stage of adolescent maturation—regularization of ovulation (1, 13, 20). Therefore, if 2 girls of the same age are similarly exposed, the more mature one is more likely to conceive.

Although the less mature girl may seem to derive a paradoxical degree of protection from her undernutrition, she is not without hazard. We have reported our analysis of data collected by the Institute of Nutrition of Central America and Panama (INCAP) in a Latin American population which strongly suggests that there exists a physiologic age threshold for optimum childbearing (23, 24, 25). Among the best nourished women, those in the 90th nutritional percentile, each year below 16 in which a woman had her first child significantly raised the risk that a surviving child under 2 years of age would show reduced height–weight attainment.

In some societies where child marriage has been the prevailing pattern, menarche has often been the signal for consummation of marriage. With the customary family pressure on the young bride for prompt motherhood, the outcome of the pregnancy is threatened or the surviving offspring is disadvantaged. In more industrialized countries, on the other hand, chronologic age is a strong determinant of sexual practice, and the early maturing female is doubly safeguarded by her better nutritional status and a longer postmenarcheal interval free from pregnancy.

DELAY OF FULL PHYSIOLOGIC MATURATION

In the meanwhile, the late maturing female is exposed to a somewhat different set of health hazards. Among the four assumptions taken, the concept of post-ovulatory optimum physiologic readiness for reproduction is more difficult to concretize physiologically than the others, although the epidemiologic evidence is appreciable. Looking at the question conceptually, and knowing that few if any endocrine organs exercise only a single specific function, it is logical to expect that a manifest deficit such as occurs in irregular ovulation is paralleled by other aberrations. For example, the pituitary's role in the great increase in blood volume that normally begins rather early in pregnancy is of particular interest in early teenage pregnancies. Furthermore, independence of a hormone's different actions occurs partially because of differential organ response readiness, and the homeostatic endocrine system more often than not precludes having only first level impact of deficits. Relevant examples are a functionally immature corpus luteum or a pituitary less responsive to the hypothalamus.

Therefore, the hypothesis is held that the late maturing female also has a longer interval between first ovulation and full reproductive maturity (1). This *vulnerable fecund interval* is prolonged because it is delayed more at the end, full maturation, than at the beginning, ovulation. According to the best data available, the menstrual pattern of females under 15 is three times as variable as that of adult women and twice as variable between 15 and 19. In one report, an anovulatory rate of 30% was still found at 18 years of age, and variability exists even among ovulatory cycles. It is interesting that the variability is largely found in the preovulatory phase of the cycle, and that the variability up to 20 years of age is almost double that of the succeeding years. The mean length of the total cycle does not shorten to, and stabilize at, the characteristic adult level for 7 years after menopause (16). Again, in most societies, there exists for the late maturing female a shorter interval between menarche and sexual exposure and correspondingly less time for optimum maturation before pregnancy.

In the study of the INCAP material just referred to, which covered a rather homogeneous social class of rural women, the data show that degrees of maternal undernutrition require progressive compensations in age above 16 years to reduce the threat of underdevelopment of the surviving young child (23). The 15½-year-old female in the 90th nutritional percentile had a chance of having a young child in best nutritional group equivalent to that of the 21-year-old woman in the 50th nutritional percentile and the 24½-year-old woman in the 10th nutritional percentile. There is a trade-off between age and nutrition. Good maternal nutrition and age above 16 years is a favorable combination. Good nutrition and younger age is unfavorable. Older age, but with poor nutrition, is disadvantageous. Poor nutrition and younger age is calamitous.

Our explanation for these phenomena rests in part on the concept of staircase-shaped nutritional thresholds, rising with age, for all three stages of reproductive development: menarche, ovulation, and maturity. Within this concept, ovulation is more easily prevented by undernutrition in the younger girl. The older girl will tolerate a greater degree of nutritional deprivation and yet begin to ovulate.

DELAYED SKELETAL GROWTH

The postmenarcheal segment of skeletal growth of the late maturing female is prolonged (2, 3, 20), with greater likelihood of overlap between continuing growth, irregular ovulation, and pregnancy. Again, there arises the concept of competition between concurrent needs, with growth favored over reproductive development, at least at first, and probably with shifting preferential use of nutrient resources with movement through the adolescent and postadolescent years.

Thus, the late maturing female suffers the fourfold threat from pregnancy, undernutrition, recent or concurrent growth, and less than optimum physiologic maturation for reproduction. These insults against her are twice further compounded. Presser (14, 15) has shown that the age of a woman at the time of birth of her first child sets for her a reproductive lifestyle of early start and many pregnancies, with concomitant family and economic implications. In addition, loss of a desired pregnancy is usually followed quickly by another pregnancy. Even in well-developed countries, the obstetrician often soothes the disappointed couple by telling them to "go home and make another baby," instead of carefully advising them to allow time for any adverse health conditions to be alleviated (7, 18). The undernourished, late maturing, but still too young mother has greater risk of a fetal or early infant death (10, 12, 17) and therefore of soon being pregnant again.

Two general objectives of program intervention are obvious: to try to prevent or overcome undernutrition among adolescent females and to avoid pregnancy at early ages. Such ambitious goals are easier stated than achieved, but may seem less unattainable if they are translated into six service elements.

1. Large scale nutrition programs, which usually give priority to pregnant women, infants, and weanlings, must consider the adolescent and preadolescent female a prime target. A particularly rigid nutritional standard should be set for the late maturing girl.

2. Contacts with the adolescents in such programs should be capitalized on to discourage early pregnancy for all early maturing females, even though well nourished, and for late maturing females during their prolonged vulnerable fecund period.

3. Promotion of good nutrition should be an essential aggressive element in the management of delayed menarche and amenorrhea in young adult women, but pregnancy should be delayed until better than marginal nutritional improvement is achieved.

4. In the presence of marked undernutrition, a woman between 16 and 20 years of age should be advised to delay pregnancy until her nutritional status is improved.

5. The care of teenage pregnancy should be characterized by nutritional protection rather than dietary restriction.

6. Unfavorable outcome of pregnancy in young women, especially when associated with undernutrition, should call for strong recommendation to delay the next pregnancy.

CONCLUSION

In the history of the evolution of medical concepts on good maternity care, stages of health supervision have been added sequentially. (Unfortunately, most women in the world do not benefit from them as yet.) The first of these was the realization that qualified attendance at childbirth is desirable; the second, that complications could be prevented by prenatal diagnosis and supervision, and the third, that a postpartum checkup helps to assess the residual gynecologic and general health status of the woman.

For many years, these constituted the recommended triad of maternity care. To a very limited degree, the postpartum examination has, in addition, become the moment for instituting continuing, preventive intergestational supervision (21) for a selected number of high risk women who are notoriously vulnerable to repetition of unfavorable outcome in successive pregnancies (7, 18).

Now we need to add to our concept and, one hopes, to our services, a fifth stage, reaching the woman before the other stages—that of preparing adolescent females for a good start in their reproductive life history.

REFERENCES

1. Baanders–Van Halewijn EA, De Waard F: Menstrual cycles shortly after menarche in European and Bantu girls. Hum Biol 40:314, 1968
2. Dreizen S, Spirakis CN, Stone RE: A comparison of skeletal growth and maturation in undernourished and well-nourished girls before and after menarche. J Pediatr 70(2):256, 1967
3. Dugdale AE, Chen ST, Hewitt G: Patterns of growth and nutrition in childhood. Am J Clin Nutr 23(1):1280, 1970
4. Frisch RE: Weight at menarche: similarity for well-nourished and under-nourished girls at differing ages, and evidence for historical constancy. Pediatrics 50(3):445, 1972
5. Frisch RE: The critical weight at menarche and the initiation of the adolescent growth spurt, and the control of puberty. In Grumbach MM, Grave GD, Mayer FE (eds): The Control of the Onset of Puberty. New York, Wiley Interstate, 1974, pp 403–423
6. Frisch RE, McArthur J: Menstrual cycles: fatness as a determinant of minimum weight for height necessary for their maintenance or onset. Science 185:949, 1974
7. Gardiner EM, Yerushalmy J: Familial susceptibility to stillbirths and neonatal deaths. Am J Epidemiol 30:11, 1939
8. Gopalan C, Nadamuni Naidu A: Nutrition and fertility. Lancet 2:1077, 1972
9. Johnston FE, Malina RM, Galbraith MA: Height, weight, and age at menarche and the "critical weight" hypothesis. Science 174:1148, 1971
10. King JC, Cohenour SH, Calloway DH, Jacobson HN: Assessment of nutritional status of teenage pregnant girls. 1. Nutrient intake and pregnancy. Am J Clin Nutr 25:916, 1972
11. Liskin B, Wishik SM: A study of nutrition states and age of menarche in 608 school girls in New Jersey. New York, International Institute for the Study of Human Reproduction, Columbia University, 1975
12. McGanity W, Little HM, Fogelman A, Jennings L, Calhour E, Dawson EB: Pregnancy in the adolescent. 1. Preliminary summary of health status. Am J Obstet Gynecol 103(6):773, 1969
13. Montague A: The Reproductive Development of the Female. Springfield, Ill, CC Thomas, 1957
14. Presser HB: The timing of the first birth, female roles and black fertility. Milbank Mem Fund Q 49(3):329, 1971
15. Presser HB: Early motherhood: ignorance or bliss? Fam Plann Perspect 6(1):8, 1974
16. Presser HB: Temporal data relating to the human menstrual cycle. In Ferin M et al. (eds): Biorhythms and Human Reproduction. A Conference Sponsored by the International Institute for the Study of Human Reproduction. New York, John Wiley & Sons, 1974, pp 145–160
17. Relation of nutrition to pregnancy in adolescence. In Maternal Nutrition and the Course of Pregnancy. Washington DC, Committee on Maternal Nutrition, National Academy of Sciences, 1970, pp 367–392
18. Schlesinger ER, Allaway N: Trends in familial susceptibility to perinatal loss. Am J Pub Health 45(2):174, 1955
19. Stein Z, Susser M: Fertility, fecundity, famine: food rations in the Dutch famine 1944/5 have a causal relation to fertility, and probably to fecundity. Hum Biol 47(1):131, 1975

20. Tanner JM: Growth at Adolescence, 2nd ed. Philadelphia, Blackwell Scientific, 1962
21. Wishik SM: How much for maternal health? Bull Maternal Welfare 5(1):11 1958
22. Wishik SM: Nutrition, family planning and fertility. Protein Group Bull 2(4):8, 1972
23. Wishik SM, Lichtblau NS: The physical development of breastfed young children as related to close birth spacing, high parity and maternal undernutrition. New York, International Institute for the Study of Human Reproduction, Columbia University, 1974
24. Wishik SM, Van der Vynckt S: Nutrition, mother's health and fertility: the effects of childbearing on health and nutrition. Background paper prepared for World Population Conference, Bucharest, Romania, August, 1974
25. Wishik SM, Van der Vynckt S: The use of nutritional "positive deviants" to identify approaches for modification of dietary practices. Am J Pub Health 66:38, 1976

Chapter 4

Nutrition in the Adolescent

William J. McGanity*

Over the past two decades we have witnessed the rise and fall of the American birth and fertility rate. With the broad-scale acceptance of family planning methods and programs, the total number of births has dropped almost 1 million per year since 1960. The current fertility rate has been hovering about 15 per thousand for the past 2 to 3 years. In truth, we are currently at zero population growth (ZPG).

There has been some unevenness in the impact that family planning programs have achieved among certain segments of our reproductive-aged population, notably among teenaged, sexually active females in minority groups. As a consequence, there has not been a significant change in the total number of live births among American young women less than 20 years of age. On a national average, they account for over 20% of all live births. On a public university hospital service such as that at the University of Texas Medical Branch in Galveston, the figure is 40% of all live births, with almost 70% of first pregnancies occurring in young women less than 20 years of age.

The nutritional consequences on the fetus of pregnancy occurring during maternal adolescence vis-á-vis the maternal nutritional consequences when pregnancy is superimposed upon adolescent growth and development have been the theses of several reports over the past two decades (1–5, 8, 9, 15, 16).

If one accepts the premise that pregnancy is a physiologic rather than pathologic state, then the preconceptional condition and preparation for childbearing may be of vital importance. While our colleagues in animal husbandry and the agrobusiness community seem to understand these propositions, this concept remains quite foreign or alien to the human counterpart—young parents.

Could it be possible that potential mothers, and even fathers, are made and nurtured from birth through childhood? If so, the growth and development during the first 17 years of life for a young woman becomes critical.

Normal biologic growth follows a very ordered series of events relating physical growth and development concomitant with endocrinologic and sexual maturation. For the female, menarche is the most important marker. Once this has occurred, only two more inches of height growth remains for the young adolescent. Caloric requirements and caloric intake during growth increase to meet the

*This work was supported in part by 5 grants and contracts from: 1) PH 86–68–123; 2) DHEW #CC/D/21; 3) OEO #CG–6805; 4) Texas Dept. of Health IAC #309; 5) NIH/NICHD #HD2–2728.

additional demands of tissue synthesis as well as physical activity. These requirements and intakes peak just prior to the onset of menarche, then rapidly decline to adult levels within the next 2 to 3 years. Growth being an anabolic process, the demands and storage of such nutritional factors as protein, calcium, and the like will parallel the caloric pattern of need and food ingestion.

NUTRITION SURVEYS OF TEXAS ADOLESCENTS

In an attempt to examine how well young women are being prepared for their first pregnancy, three unpublished studies originating from our group* at the University of Texas Medical Branch, Galveston, are presented. The data are based on the following cross-sectional and longitudinal projects:

1. Cross-sectional data on approximately 1300 youngsters who participated in the Texas Nutrition Survey (TNS) during the years 1968 and 1969. Their ages ranged from 0–16 years, and they were derived from lower income Mexican-American, black, and white populations.
2. Longitudinal and cross-sectional data from four separate studies performed on over 2000 children enrolled in school-sponsored educational and feeding programs. Their ages ranged from 2–16 years and they were from the three major ethnic clusters of the population of Texas.
3. Longitudinal data obtained from 93 young women less than 25 years of age who were utilizing one or another form of oral contraceptive agents.

In each study, we used the procedures and methods developed for the Ten State Nutrition Survey (NNS) and utilized their standards of *low* and *deficient* where applicable (14).

The population sample for the NNS was of a three-step, random-sample design and was drawn from population groups who resided in the lower economic quartile areas of each state. Two different economic clusters of states resulted: 1) Those with a low mean poverty index ratio (PIR) of about 1.1. Texas data fell into this group, with 60% of the families having a PIR of less than 1.0 and an average family of four having a mean annual income in 1968 of just over $3400. 2) High-income states with a mean PIR of 1.8. The Michigan sample was included in this group, with 28% of the families having a PIR of less than 1.0 and the average family of four receiving a mean annual income of almost $7800.

The resultant population seen in the Texas Nutrition Survey comprised predominantly minority subjects—46% Mexican-Americans, 39% blacks, and 15% whites. There was a considerable lack of formal education of either heads of households and/or their spouses, more so in Mexican-American families than

*Over the past 5 years encompassed by 4 of the studies, our group included over 35 professional qualified individuals of whom 20 were medical students (now graduated physicians), 5 nutritionists and home economists, 5 biochemists, 3 statisticians, and 2 anthropometrists. During the Texas Nutrition Survey of 1968–69, our team included an additional 25 professional and 63 allied health members.

in the black or white families. Overall, 10% of the family heads had received no formal education at all, a third had completed less than the sixth grade level, and only 5% had progressed beyond grade 12.

When the nutritional and medical histories of the present preschool and school-aged children are evaluated, one is surprised to learn of some of the obstacles they have already overcome. Our TNS sample included 797 reproductive-aged women who had had almost 4400 pregnancies. One in five had become pregnant prior to age 17 and 52% before age 20. Overall reproductive failure amounted to 26%. Low-birth-weight infants were born at a rate 1% greater than either the current national or state frequency (9.2% versus 8.2% of live births). The perinatal and infant mortality rates of 78 and 57 per 1000 live births were two to three times higher than data from either Texas or the United States. So, for these children to even reach age 1 year required hurdling several obstacles.

Table 4–1 presents a few items of the children's past and current medical profiles, which reflects higher rates of breast-feeding than in the general American population and a considerable lack of preventive medical and dental health care. It is no wonder that the state of dentition was a disaster, as can be seen from Table 4–6.

Turning to more traditional evidence of nutritional assessment, the dietary intake of the children in the TNS sample revealed significant and consistent evidence of the participants having an inadequate food intake. Based on the 24-hour dietary recall method (Table 4–2) and measured against the NNS nutrient intake standard, the data showed that 13–69% of the infants, 7–28% of the teenagers, and 12–52% of the pregnant and/or lactating mothers failed to ingest 50% of the reference nutrient standard. The NNS nutrient standard was identical to the 1968 Recommended Dietary Allowances of the National Research Council except for the lower NNS Standards for the intake of calcium and vitamins A and C (14).

Is it any wonder that we found growth retardation in our TNS sample of

Table 4–1. PERCENT OF CHILDREN IN TEXAS NUTRITION SURVEY (1968) WITH POSITIVE HISTORIES OF SELECTED MEDICAL CONDITIONS

| | | 6–16 yrs. | |
	0–5 yrs	Females	Males
Breast-fed	27%		
Completed immunization	33%–51%		
Passed worms prior 6 months	5%		
Ingested various forms Pica	12%	12%*	
Never seen a dentist	95%	65%*	
Prior major surgery	1%	3%	4%
Family history of diabetes		14%	12%
Positive medical history of:			
Anemia		3%	1%
Allergies		7%	6%
Treatment for obesity		1%	1%
Renal disease		2%	1%
Fractures		1%	3%

*Combined male and female value.

Table 4–2. PERCENTAGE OF INFANTS, TEENAGERS, AND PREGNANT AND/OR LACTATING WOMEN IN TEXAS NUTRITION SURVEY (1968) INGESTING LESS THAN FIFTY PERCENT OF NUTRIENT STANDARD, AS MEASURED BY THE 24-HOUR RECALL METHOD

	0–3 yrs (N=110)	10–16 yrs (N=822)	P/L* (N=35)
Calories	22%	13%	32%
Protein	13%	7%	23%
Calcium	24%	26%	43%
Iron	69%	26%	34%
Vitamin A	23%	17%	52%
Vitamin C	49%	20%	26%
Thiamine	16%	14%	17%
Riboflavin	14%	15%	12%
Niacin	34%	28%	20%

*Pregnant and lactating

Fig. 4–1. Comparative height-weight data for girls to 6 years of age, Texas Nutrition Survey (1968). The standard is that of H. V. Meredith, Iowa Child Research Station (copyrighted 1943).

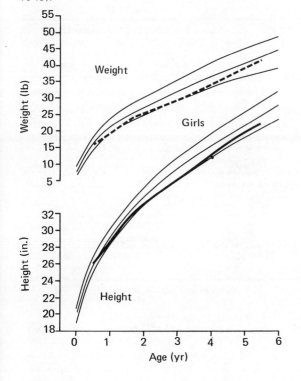

children (Fig. 4–1, Tables 3 and 4). Comparison of mean height growth of the preschooler (Fig. 4–1) against the Meredith-Iowa Growth Curve has revealed a rate of growth that falls along the 16th rather than the 50th percentile line. Translated into absolute terms, the children were 1 inch shorter than "normal American children" by age 3 years. Our later cross-sectional sample data indicate that this deficit is never made up. Analysis of the data by family PIR and ethnic background (Table 4–3) demonstrates that height growth retardation of less than one standard deviation is more likely when the PIR is lowest and that it is more common in the Mexican-American child than in either the black or white child of age 0–6 years. With the increased frequency of "low" levels of four blood or urinary nutrients (Table 4–4) among preschoolers with less than one standard deviation in height growth retardation in the TNS sample, it seems apparent that there may even be a nutritional deficiency component to the height growth retardation we found in these subjects. Comparison of these data to those obtained from children of similar age in developing countries overseas

Table 4–3. PERCENTAGE OF 0- TO 6-YEAR-OLD CHILDREN IN TEXAS NUTRITION SURVEY (1968) WITH LOW HEIGHT AND WEIGHT STATUS BY POVERTY INDEX RATIO (PIR) AND ETHNIC GROUP

PIR		Percent low height*				Percent low weight†		
	Total‡	Mexican-American	Black	White	Total§	Mexican-American	Black	White
< 0.5	46	55	33	—	46	51	40	42
0.5–0.99	43	52	32	33	48	50	46	60
1.0–1.49	39	35	43	50	47	44	48	—
≥ 1.5	25	17	30	—	23	22	31	—
Total‖	43	51	33	38	46	49	44	43

*Values lower than 1 standard deviation below the average of the Iowa Growth Standard.
†Values lower than the 16th percentile of the Iowa Growth Standard.
‡Percent low height by income regardless of ethnic group.
§Percent low weight by income regardless of ethnic group.
‖Percent low weight and height regardless of income and ethnic group.

Table 4–4. PERCENTAGE OF 0- TO 6-YEAR-OLD PARTICIPANTS IN THE TEXAS NUTRITION SURVEY MANIFESTING GROWTH RETARDATION, LOW WEIGHT, AND LOW BIOCHEMICAL VALUES

Measurement	Percent low values in group		
	Low biochemical values	Low height*	Low weight†
Hemoglobin	6	6	5
Serum albumin	4	11	10
Plasma vitamin C	21	29	27
Plasma vitamin A	32	41	41
Urinary thiamine	5	4	3
Urinary riboflavin	31	36	31

*Values lower than 1 standard deviation below the average of the Iowa Growth Standard.
†Values lower than the 16th percentile of the Iowa Growth Standard.

indicates that the growth retardation in our sample is at the rate of 6 to 9 months rather than the 18 to 24 months found, for example, in the Central American Nutrition Surveys (13). Careful and detailed cross analyses of the TNS data reveal that the growth retardation is for height and bone age only and not for weight. When one compares data for height to data for weight within age groupings, the apparent weight retardation seen in Figure 4–1 and Tables 4–3 and 4–4 disappears.

As the youngsters progress through the school years, their patterns of height and weight growth change (Fig. 4–2). Mean height moves up along the 30–40% line, and mean weight begins to increase around the prepubertal spurt, so much so that weight crosses the 50th percentile and does not stop going up after female growth maturation is reached at age 17 years. At that age, 14% of the young women were more than 120% of standard weight. By age 35 years, over 50% of the women in the TNS sample were obese. So we have height growth retardation at one stage and overt obesity at another.

From the over 30 clinical manifestations of nutritional disorders that were assessed, Table 4–5 presents eight of the indicator signs that were used in the TNS data. These were evidence of mild to moderate nutritional insufficiency rather than frank deficiency disease. However, we did find 4 cases of classic protein-caloric malnutrition in our sample. The incidence of physical signs in

Fig. 4–2 Comparative height-weight data for girls ages 5–10 years, Texas Nutrition Survey (1968). The standard is that of H. V. Meredith, Iowa Child Research Station (copyrighted 1943).

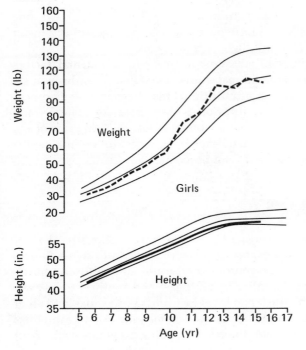

this table are eight to ten times what one would anticipate in a nutritionally healthy American population.

As pointed out earlier in Table 4–1, preventive and/or crisis dental care was not utilized or available to the vast majority of growing children in the Texas sample. Home dental care—as reflected by having and/or utilizing a toothbrush on at least a daily basis—provided equally dismal data (Table 4–6). Is it any wonder that the average 10- to 16-year-old had almost six cavities, that over 90% of the young people were in need of a filling, and that in one-quarter of the instances the disease process had gone so far that dental extraction of a permanent tooth was the only therapeutic solution. A major portion of the communities in Texas have natural fluoridation approaching levels that protect against dental decay. In such areas, the children in our TNS sample had 30% fewer cavities in spite of no dental hygiene or care.

Depending on the nutrient assayed, from 700 to 900 aliquots of blood and urine were available for the over 20 biochemical nutrients measured from the TNS sample of children. Data on the percent "low" or at-risk population of children in the TNS sample for seven essential nutrient factors are presented in Table 4–7. Trends were observed with advancing age in the mean levels of several of these nutrients—hemoglobin and vitamins A and C—which are not presented but were incorporated into the standards of "low" utilized in the NNS. From 10–38% of the children of 0–16 years of age were at risk in one nutrient factor or another. When these are all combined into a comprehensive biochemical index (Table 4–8) we find that there was a significant percentage (24–41%) of both girls and boys in the Texas sample that were seriously at risk, having two or more "low" biochemical levels in the same individual. When one compares Texas data with similar items from the other Ten State Surveys, one finds the same pattern of "2+ low" biochemistry levels with age but at a lower level of magnitude with the low and high income status.

In summation: Ethnic, economic, educational, medical, and dental factors were found to influence apparent nutritional assessment. Dietary, anthropometric, clinical, and biochemical evidence of nutritional insufficiency and its consequences were present in the Texas Nutrition Survey data for children and adolescents. Is it any wonder that the young woman of less than 20 years of age enters her first pregnancy with several handicaps in her quest for optimal reproductive performance and maternal and fetal outcome.

SCHOOL FEEDING PROGRAMS

During 1970–1972, we monitored, prospectively and cross-sectionally, the nutritional status of over 2100 preschool and school-aged students (Table 4–9) who were enrolled in four public-school-sponsored educational health and nutritional projects in four different counties in southeast and southcentral Texas. Each of the projects had school lunch and breakfast programs available to all of the children for at least the traditional 9-month school year. All 16 samplings were carried out during the time when the school feeding programs were about to begin or were in force.

Table 4–5. PERCENT OF SUBJECTS IN TEXAS NUTRITION SURVEY (1968) WITH CLINICAL SIGNS OF NUTRITIONAL DEFICIENCY BY AGE

Deficient nutrient(s)	Clinical sign	0–6 yrs.	6–16 yrs	16+ yrs
Protein/Calorie	Abnormal hair (color/texture)	2.1%	0.6%	0.3%
Iron or B vitamins	Filiform papillary atrophy	3.3%	4.4%	6.2%
Vitamin A	Follicular hyperkeratosis	3.1%	4.9%	3.9%
Vitamin D	Enlarged wrists	2.8%	—	—
Vitamin C	Swollen, red gums	0.6%	5.9%	8.5%
Riboflavin	Angular lesions of tongue;	1.4%	0.9%	0.6%
	glossitis of tongue	0.4%	2.0%	8.3%
Iodine	Visible enlargement of thyroid	1.1%	5.4%	5.5%

Table 4–6. PERCENT OF SCHOOL-AGED CHILDREN IN TEXAS NUTRITION SURVEY (1968) WITH SELECTED DENTAL FINDINGS IN PERMANENT TEETH BY AGE

	5–9 yrs	10–16 yrs
Total with decayed, missing, and filled teeth	4.3%	7.5%
Decayed	1.0%	5.9%
Missing	0.5%	1.1%
Filled	0.5%	0.5%
Peridontal disease	5.4%	22.5%
Need fillings	87.4%	91.5%
Need extractions	34.6%	25.2%

Table 4–7. PERCENT OF CHILDREN IN TEXAS NUTRITION SURVEY (1968–1969) WITH "LOW" BIOCHEMISTRY BY AGE

	Age (yrs)				
	0–5	6–9	10–12	13–16	0–16
Serum albumin	5.1%	12.0%	10.3%	15.8%	12.1%
Hemoglobin	8.6%	7.9%	7.7%	11.5%	9.1%
Hematocrit	12.7%	17.2%	8.8%	11.5%	12.8%
Serum iron	1.0%	3.4%	0.0%	0.0%	3.3%
Serum vitamin A	45.6%	41.8%	39.9%	29.2%	37.9%
Serum vitamin C	9.3%	9.0%	13.2%	13.0%	11.6%
Urinary thiamine	2.6%	11.7%	12.4%	10.8%	9.9%
Urinary riboflavin	29.7%	31.3%	22.5%	32.1%	28.9%

Table 4–8. PERCENT OF CHILDREN IN TEXAS NUTRITION SURVEY (1968) WITH "2+ LOW" BIOCHEMICAL INDEX BY AGE, SEX, AND INCOME STATUS

	Sex		Income Status*	
Age	Males	Females	Low	High
0–5 yrs	31%	41%	24%	3%
6–9 yrs	32%	31%	25%	5%
10–12 yrs	32%	24%	} 23%	} 7%
13–16 yrs	36%	35%		

*Low as defined by NNS Standard; income status groupings of Ten State Nutrition Survey Data.

Table 4–9. PERCENT OF CHILDREN IN FOUR TEXAS STUDIES (1970–1972) WITH "LOW" BIO-CHEMISTRY

	Study				
	ECLC-I	ECLC-II	Newton	Goiter	Combined
Year(s)	1970–1972	1970–1972	1970–1972	1972	1970–1972
Number of samplings	6	4	4	2	16
Age (yrs)	2–5	2–5	6–16	10–16	2–16
Number of subjects	321	269	1211	319	2120
Children with					
"low" Hb (%)	12.5	12.3	7.9	0.7	8.1
Serum vitamin A (%)	25.9	37.5	11.2	38.6	20.9
Serum vitamin C (%)	2.2	0.7	0.3	0.0	0.6
Urinary thiamine (%)	6.2	11.5	26.8	17.9	20.4
Urinary riboflavin (%)	27.7	25.7	20.0	15.0	21.1
Children with					
"2+ low" index (%)			26.7	16.3	

ECLC, Early Childhood Learning Center; Hb, hemoglobin.

The overall percentage of children with "low" at-risk biochemical nutrients (Table 4–9) reveals an absence of any problems with vitamin C. However, 1 in 5 of the students were assessed as being at risk with respect to their vitamin A, thiamine, and riboflavin status. "Low" hemoglobin values varied with the age and location of the study group(s). Similar to data presented above for youngsters in the TNS who had two or more "low" biochemical values, two of the school feeding program studies revealed that one-sixth to one-fourth of the subjects were also at serious nutritional risk when one utilized similar criteria. The Early Childhood Learning Center (ECLC) projects involved two subsets of participants and feeding phases of their program (Tables 4–9 to 4–12).

ECLC-I children were predominately Mexican-American and white students enrolled in a bilingual enrichment program developed and operated by the local public school system. The program commenced in September 1970 and has been expanded over the past 5 years. We monitored it nutritionally over the first 2 years. The school feeding phase involved both breakfast and lunch served to all children in the classroom under direct supervision of the homeroom teacher. The program was active from 7:30 A.M. to 2:30 P.M., 5 days a week during the school year, September through May.

ECLC-II children were predominantly black and white students at the same center with an added late afternoon day care component. The program began in April 1971. It still exists in an expanded format now in several locations in the community. The school feeding included breakfast, lunch, and a late afternoon snack for all student participants. The program was active throughout the calendar year, 5 days a week from 7:00 A.M. to 6:00 P.M. Both programs included preventive health and dental care, education of parents and teachers about nutrition, as well as the school feeding portion. Qualified nutritionists worked on site in food planning and preparation and in the nutritional education effort oriented towards the parents, classroom teachers, center administrators, and—in very simple show-and-tell type efforts—the children themselves. Our study was prospective in design, following serially students enrolled in the ECLC over the 2-year period.

Environmental variations between the two groups in the project are illustrated in Table 4–10, with the bilingual youngsters coming from a Spanish-speaking background of somewhat higher economic status than the Day Care children.

Visible improvement in the health and nutritional status of the children was evident within 6 months of their participation, as revealed by a height/weight growth increment that was at a more rapid rate than anticipated for average American children of similar age and the complete disappearance of any clinical manifestation of nutritional insufficiency.

Supporting biochemical nutritional data (Tables 4–11 and 4–12) was evident for both groups when evaluated for percent of children with "low" levels of serum albumin and hemoglobin whether analyzed by season (Table 4–11) or by time in program (Table 4–12). Similar improvement was found with thiamine status as reflected by urinary excretion. Riboflavin nutriture tended to improve during the first 8 months and in the spring of 1972.

The explanation of the variations in vitamin C status during the first 8 months of the study may in small part have been due to seasonal availability of the nutrient from food. The major reason, we believe, was the former rules and regulations for the use of school breakfast foods which required that all items must be provided at one sitting in the morning. The small stomachs of 2- to 4-year-olds could not cope with all the cereal, milk, and fruit juice. Something had to give way! It was the fruit juice. In the spring of 1971 we received permission to change the time when the fruit juice was offered until just before going home in the early afternoon. The mean serum vitamin C levels were quickly doubled, and the "low" at-risk category disappeared.

The vitamin A story was a magnificent failure. Dark green and yellow vegetables were not selling to mother, teacher, or preschool child. The marked increase in "low" serum levels of vitamin A in the second year of the program we attribute to the in-service training provided the classroom teachers by a "nutritionally renowned" behavioral psychologist. As everyone should know, children left to their own devices will naturally select the correct food items, when offered, to meet their own nutrient requirements! The results speak for themselves during both 1972 samplings: mean serum vitamin A levels in the two groups were under 20 μg/100 ml.

While considerable benefit was evident for the children, it appears that some other way needs to be found to get adequate amounts of vitamin A into such children. Would not low-fat milk enriched with both vitamins A and D be a better nutritional choice than old-fashioned Grade A homogenized milk?

The Newton Study in rural deep east Texas (Tables 4–9, and 4–13 to 4–17) was prospective and also involved elementary and junior high school children aged 6–16 years, in grades K through 8. They were almost equally black and white. Their families' mean PIR was approximately 1.5. The area itself is in the "Piney Wood" section of Texas, and lumbering is the major industry. Environmental characteristics (Table 4–13) revealed that the home food intake was augmented in many families by having home gardens and chickens.

Table 4–10. PERCENT OF CHILDREN IN EARLY CHILDHOOD PROGRAMS (1970–1972) WITH SELECTED HOME ENVIRONMENTAL CHARACTERISTICS

Families that	Bilingual	Day care
Own home	50%	4%
Live in public housing	10%	28%
Speak Spanish in home	24%	5%
Receive food commodities	7%	42%

Table 4–11. PERCENT OF CHILDREN IN EARLY CHILDHOOD PROGRAMS (1970–1972) WITH "LOW" BIOCHEMISTRY BY SEASON

		1970		1971		1972	
		Fall	Winter	Spring	Fall	Spring	Fall
Number of children	Bil	60	65	62	42	43	49
	DC			37	93	89	50
Percent of children with deficiency in							
Serum albumin	Bil	11	7	16	0	3	0
	DC			4	4	2	0
Hemoglobin	Bil	12	0	21	0	0	0
	DC			68	4	1	6
Serum vitamin A	Bil	6	12	17	30	46	55
	DC			24	21	50	54
Serum vitamin C	Bil	0	8	4	0	0	0
	DC			6	0	0	0
Urinary riboflavin	Bil	27	39	16	11	9	59
	DC			28	25	7	47

Bil, bilingual enrichment program; DC, day care program.

Table 4–12. PERCENT OF CHILDREN IN EARLY CHILDHOOD PROGRAMS (1970–1972) WITH "LOW" BIOCHEMISTRY BY TIME IN PROGRAM

		Months				
		0	4	8	12	18
Number of children	Bil	106	83	42	31	39
	DC	99		83	65	12
Percent of children with deficiency in						
Serum albumin	Bil	7	12	10	0	0
	DC	4		4	0	0
Hemoglobin	Bil	7	10	10	3	3
	DC	25		4	5	9
Serum vitamin A	Bil	10	21	20	43	59
	DC	22		43	51	58
Serum vitamin C	Bil	1	5	5	0	0
	DC	2		0	0	0
Urinary riboflavin	Bil	22	29	14	18	21
	DC	26		12	32	54

Bil, bilingual enrichment program; DC, day care program.

Table 4–13. PERCENT OF CHILDREN (N = 1310) IN RURAL TEXAS SCHOOL PROGRAM (1970–1971) WITH SELECTED HOME ENVIRONMENTAL CHARACTERISTICS

Families that	Percent children
Own home	60
Use well water	20
Have:	
Home garden	54
Farm animals	42
Adequate refrigeration	98
Working television	93

Table 4–14. PERCENT OF CHILDREN (IN GRADES K–8) IN RURAL TEXAS SCHOOL PROGRAM (1970–1971) WITH CERTAIN DIETARY CHARACTERISTICS

	Nov. 1970	May 1971
Never eat		
Breakfast	8%	8%
Between meals	13%	11%
Eat		
School breakfast 5 ×/wk	87%	84%
School lunch 5 ×/wk	76%	95%
Use		
Free breakfast	91%	82%
Free lunch	19%	46%
Pica		3%
Daily Mineral/vitamin		20%
Daily—junk food		20–40%

Table 4–15. MEAN INCREASE IN HEIGHT AND WEIGHT PER YEAR IN NINE- TO TEN-YEAR-OLD CHILDREN IN RURAL TEXAS SCHOOL PROGRAM (1970–1971)

	Height increase (cm)			Weight increase (kg)		
	Nov. 1970 (9)	May 1971 (9.5)	Nov. 1971 (10)	Nov. 1970 (9)	May 1971 (9.5)	Nov. 1971 (10)
Males						
White	0	2.1	7.5	0	1.0	4.3
Black	0	2.5	6.7	0	1.4	3.4
50° Standards*	0	—	4.8	0	—	2.7
Females						
White	0	2.2	6.6	0	0.9	3.0
Black	0	2.4	6.7	0	1.9	5.2
50° Standards*	0	—	5.7	0	—	3.0

*Stuart–Meredith Standards. Age in years given in parentheses.

Children in the three schools in the two school districts were studied over a 12-month period during 1970–1971. During the first 6 months, they were all provided a free school breakfast in addition to the available school lunch which was a standardized fare of food based on the menus provided from the state education agency. There was no nutritional input into local menu planning, let alone any nutritional requirements built into their local food purchases.

Table 4–14 provides an insight into the dietary practices of these children during the 6-month feeding trial period.

It was discouraging that the average student spent 30 cents per day on "junk food", with 30% of the children purchasing potato chips, 20–40% bought candy, 35% soda pop and 20% pastries. It was equally disappointing to find the vending machines selling these "junk foods" located either in the school cafeteria or in the corridor outside the principal's office.

In spite of the above shortcomings, the rates of height and weight growth over the year for the children of both sexes and color exceeded prediction (Table 4–15). There was lower than expected incidence of height and weight retardation (Table 4–16) coupled with an excess abundance of obesity among the female and white male subjects.

From the nutritional biochemical viewpoint (Table 4–17), the vitamin A and C nutriture was quite satisfactory. We have no ready explanation of the ups and downs of the hemoglobin, serum albumin, urinary thiamine, and riboflavin statuses during the year of serial observations in the over 300 study participants. It appears that the overall 2+ low biochemical index was lower in the fall than

Table 4–16. PERCENT OF CHILDREN IN RURAL TEXAS SCHOOL PROGRAM (MAY 1971) WITH EXTREMES OF HEIGHT AND WEIGHT WHEN COMPARED TO MEREDITH-IOWA GROWTH CHART

| | Height | Weight | |
	< 1 SD	< 16°	> 84°
Males			
White	18%	13%	26%
Black	8%	11%	14%
Females			
White	18%	12%	25%
Black	7%	8%	28%

Table 4–17. PERCENT OF CHILDREN IN RURAL TEXAS SCHOOL PROGRAM (1970–1971) WITH "LOW" BIOCHEMISTRY BY SEASON

	Nov 1970 (N=362)	May 1971 (N=402)	Nov 1971 (N=320)
Serum albumin	13%	10%	1%
Hemoglobin	3%	10%	13%
Serum vitamin A	6%	3%	5%
Serum vitamin C	0%	1%	0%
Urinary thiamine	15%	37%	25%
Urinary riboflavin	40%	41%	17%
With 0 "low" index	46%	30%	48%
With 2+ "low" index	16%	39%	23%

in the spring, due in large part to contribution of the increased number of "low" levels of hemoglobin and urinary thiamine found in subjects at the May 1971 examinations.

These observations indicate an adequate intake of calories, vitamins A and C, and probably, protein by the children during the year of study. Nutrient problems at the biochemical level of detection are present for thiamine and riboflavin among a significant number of the program participants. Could these problems be "cured" by requiring that only enriched flour, bread, and cereal products be purchased or provided in the school lunch and breakfast programs?

As a follow up to the initial NNS findings of visibly and palpably enlarged thyroid glands (goiter) among a surprising number of adolescent subjects, very detailed thyroid function studies were developed in Michigan, Kentucky, Georgia, and Texas (11, 12). In the Texas sample, over 2800 11- through 16-year-old adolescents in two widely separated counties were examined for evidence of thyroid enlargement. Goiters were found among 4.5–7.5% of the males and 8.2–9.0% of the females. Thyroid function studies demonstrated that the goiters found were not due to an iodine intake deficit.

We added a biochemical nutritional assessment to every tenth nongoitrous subject and to every subject with thyroid enlargement. Each such participant was enrolled in public school junior and senior high programs and had available a school lunch program. The location A sample was from children of middle income families with mean PIR over 2.0 within a mixed Mexican-American and white student body. The sample from location B was almost equally black and white with a lower mean income (PIR < 1.5).

Dietary intake evaluation was limited to those foods which provide significant iodine ingestion because of either natural, enriched, or processing-added content. The most important of these are listed in Table 4–18 by percent frequency of daily food use. Note the high rates of "never use" for fish and two sources of vitamin A.

The "low" biochemical nutrient profile and index (Table 4–19) revealed the same problem area described above for vitamin A, thiamine, and riboflavin. The more seriously at-risk students—those having a 2+ "low" index—occurred more in female groups and were almost three times more prevalent among our study population in location B.

The final bits of data are presented in Table 4–20 for the over 4200 children 0–19 years of age who were examined in a general population probability sample from Nutrition Canada (6). There are some similarities in the percent at "moderate biochemical risk" between the Canadian and Texas data for vitamin A and thiamine. It appears that there is more of a vitamin C problem among the Canadian youngsters, while their riboflavin nutriture is superior to that of the Texas children.

These five studies all lead to the same conclusion—that there are a significant percentage of young female children and adolescents who enter their years of reproductive capability in compromised nutritional health. Such young women are in no condition to superimpose a pregnancy upon their deficit-financed nutrient reserves.

IMPACT OF OVULATORY CONTROL AGENTS ON NUTRITIONAL STATUS

Over the past 5 years, many groups have examined the interrelationship of one or another form of ovulatory control agents (OCA) on a large number of individual macro and trace nutrients. The state of knowledge was well summarized in 1969–1972 (7, 10). At that time, many gaps were present in our knowledge of the effects of sex steroids from either endogenous or exogenous source on amino acids, lipids, metals, and water-soluble and fat-soluble vitamins. To fill in some

Table 4–18. PERCENT OF 10- TO 16-YEAR-OLDS IN TEXAS GOITER STUDY (1972) WITH SELECTED IODINE-RELATED DIETARY PRACTICES

	Two or more uses/day	Never use
Milk	44%	4%
Eggs	3%	10%
Fish	0%	32%
Meat	66%	0%
Cereals	0%	49%
Bread	74%	0%
Spinach	8%	36%
Turnips	0%	62%
Other vegetables	6%	4%
Mineral/vitamin pill	—	83%

Table 4–19. PERCENT OF 10- TO 16-YEAR-OLDS IN TEXAS GOITER STUDY (1972) WITH "LOW" BIOCHEMISTRY

	Location A		Location B	
	Females	Males	Females	Males
Serum albumin	1%	1%	4%	0%
Hemoglobin	0%	1%	0%	2%
Serum vitamin A	22%	24%	65%	66%
Serum vitamin C	0%	0%	0%	0%
Urinary thiamine	17%	5%	30%	22%
Urinary riboflavin	22%	16%	8%	8%
With 0 "low" index	51%	59%	25%	24%
With 2+ "low" index	11%	6%	31%	22%

Table 4–20. PERCENT OF GENERAL POPULATION IN NUTRITION CANADA STUDY (1970–1972) WITH "MODERATE RISK" BIOCHEMISTRY

	0–4 yrs Combined	5–9 yr Combined	10–19 yrs		15–45 yrs Pregnant females*
			Females	Males	
Hemoglobin	4.4%	4.0%	2.6%	5.8%	27.9%
Serum vitamin A	23.0%	15.3%	5.8%	4.5%	5.1%
Serum vitamin C	19.8%	17.0%	27.5%	30.5%	10.8%
Urinary thiamine	0.5%	1.8%	16.6%	10.3%	2.0%
Urinary riboflavin	3.7%	1.6%	9.4%	3.9%	2.9%

*Not probability sample.

of these gaps, our group in Galveston, the Tulane group in New Orleans, and the Wayne State University Group in Detroit have become involved in a cooperative three-part comprehensive program examining the impact of OCA use on the nutritional status of users of OCAs. To illustrate the interaction of drugs and nutritional status, our studies on these agents provide several aspects of potential hazard to the adolescent. Only one of three phases of our data, which we have accumulated over the past 3 years, will be presented.

Over 90 young women, 25 years or younger, who had less than two previous pregnancies and were not lactating have been serially assessed at 90-day intervals for over a year. Initial evaluation was performed prior to their using OCAs. Our sample was almost equally white and black, with a mean PIR of 0.9. Eighty-six percent were less than 20 years of age, 82% had never been pregnant, and 68% were less than 20 years of age and had never been pregnant. All were using one of three forms of OCA, two of which were a combined form of estrogen and progestin, the other an estrogen/progestin sequential: 39% used Ovral 21 (0.05 mg ethinyl estradiol and 0.5 mg norgestrel), a combination OCA; 24% used Norinyl 1/50–21 (0.05 mg mestranol and 1 mg norethindrone), a combination OCA; and 37% used Oracon–21, an ethinyl estradiol/dimethisterone sequential OCA.

Dietary intake was determined utilizing a food frequency use approach based on 33 food items which we have developed. Mean nutrient intakes of these young women exceeded the NRC and NNS recommended standards.

Over 30 biochemical parameters related to nutrition were measured serially in each subject at the initiation of OCA use and on four occasions during the subsequent year. Data for 24 of the items are presented in Table 4–21 as they existed about two-thirds of the way along the project time. From these data we can see certain trends developing.

At least two of the six nutrients we have examined so far have statistically significant differences in their levels according to the duration and type of the pill used.

1. There was a progressive increase with time of use of the ovulatory control agent of serum levels of iron, cholesterol, and α-globulin, and of vitamin B_6 activity and urinary iron excretion.

2. There was a progressive decrease with time of OCA use of serum levels of albumin, magnesium, and triglycerides, and in RBC folate of urinary excretion of riboflavin.

3. There were some nutrients whose levels fluctuated over the first year of observation. There was an initial decrease with later increase or plateau of serum levels of vitamins E and B_{12}, zinc and also of urinary zinc and copper excretion. There was an initial increase with later decrease or plateau of serum levels of vitamin A and copper and also of urinary calcium excretion.

RBC folate and serum cholesterol levels appear to be significantly influenced by the type of estrogen/progestin content of the OCA used (Table 4–22). After 9 months of OCA use, the RBC folate values had been suppressed 29% in Ovral

Table 4–21. MEAN VALUES OF BIOCHEMICAL PARAMETERS MEASURED IN WOMEN IN OVULA-
TORY CONTROL AGENT STUDY (1972–1974) AT COMMENCEMENT OF USE AND AT
3-MONTH INTERVALS THEREAFTER

	Month				
	0 (93)	3 (65)	6 (51)	9 (39)	12 (28)
Serum albumin (g/dl)	4.4	4.1	4.1	4.2	4.1
Serum α_1 globulin (g/dl)	0.23	0.28	0.28	0.28	0.31
Hemoglobin (g/dl)	13.1	13.0	12.8	12.7	12.8
Serum iron (μg/dl)	66	66	85	86	94
Serum B_{12} (ng/dl)	0.6	0.5	0.4	0.4	0.6
Serum folate (ng/dl)	5.2	5.1	5.3	5.0	2.7
RBC folate (ng/ml)	216	198	177	162	143
Serum vitamin C (mg/dl)	0.9	1.1	1.0	1.1	1.1
B_6–GOT coefficient (units/dl)	1.25	1.21	1.36	1.37	1.46
Urinary: Thiamine μg/gCr	731	410	562	305	955
Riboflavin μg/gCr	544	426	329	93	336
N1 methyl Nicotinamide μg/gCr	11.5	17.8	14.9	12.6	18.6
Serum vitamin A (μg/dl)	36	45	49	45	42
vitamin E (μg/dl)	908	849	717	883	1031
Cholesterol (mg/dl)	148	162	182	191	193
Triglyceride (mg/dl)	97	90	84	80	89
Serum: Zinc (μg/dl)	82	80	80	100	104
Copper (μg/dl)	119	161	164	128	122
Magnesium (mg/dl)	1.9	1.9	1.8	1.7	1.7
Calcium (mg/dl)	10.0	10.2	10.2	10.0	9.7
Urinary iron (mm/mCr)	470	1549	1924	2024	3640
Zinc (mm/mCr)	1416	476	344	332	458
Copper (mm/mCr)	469	122	156	166	222
Calcium (mm/mCr)	98	216	199	229	209

Number of samples are given in parentheses.

Table 4–22. ALTERATIONS WITH TIME AND MEDICATION IN UNIVERSITY OF TEXAS MEDICAL
BRANCH-OCA STUDY (1972–1974)

		Months of use				
	OCA used	0	3	6	9	12
Red cell folate (ng/dl)	Norinyl	212	199	139	119	100
	Ovral	220	218	214	157	170
	Oracon	182	143	158	103	
Serum cholesterol (mg/dl)	Norinyl	147	175	181	218	226
	Ovral	121	124	164	160	156
	Oracon	139	158	177	193	184

users and 44% in Oracon and Norinyl users. In the same time interval, serum
cholesterol levels were driven up 32% with Ovral, 38% with Oracon, and 48%
with Norinyl use.

Are these alterations a potential nutritional health hazard? Table 4–23 presents
the at-risk biochemical characteristics for 13 of the nutrients. The folate, vitamin
E, cholesterol, and riboflavin data suggest progressive deterioration with time of
pill use for these nutrients while serum iron and vitamin A findings reflect
improvement with time.

CONCLUSION

Nutrition during adolescence should result in the final maturation of biologic growth and development. However, nutritional problems from birth through the teens are only a part of the total milieu which involves the interaction of environmental, socioeconomic, educational, health, and iatrogenic influences. We have tried to illustrate this with the three major areas of data presented.

We have expanded and improved the physical growth of our adolescents in many ways over the last two generations. Have we done as well from the more strict nutritional point of view? In some ways, yes; some, no; and some, maybe. Many questions still remain.

By whom and where is the adolescent fed? The home? The school? The corner store?

Who has the most influence on the food habits and practices of the adolescent? The mother? The coach? School peers? Certainly it is not the physician.

Should school administrative officials be required to build in nutrient specifications prior to putting food purchases out for bid?

Can we ever really expect a functional nutrition education program at the school level without a requirement for at least basic nutritional courses for all education and physical health majors in teacher preparation programs at the university level?

Is there not a place for the adolescent to join with others in the food and nutritional planning of school lunch and breakfast programs? In this day of consumerism, does not the adolescent need to be represented?

Can school-based vending machines be converted to dispense nutritional food rather than junk food and still make a profit? When 15% of the schools in a large metropolitan school district in our state earn more than $100,000 profit per year

Table 4–23. PERCENT "LOW" OR "HIGH" BIOCHEMISTRY BY TIME IN UNIVERSITY OF TEXAS MEDICAL BRANCH–OCA STUDY 1972–1974

	Months	0	3	6	9	12
	N=	93	65	51	39	28
	STD used			Percent		
Serum Albumin	<3.5 g/dl	0	0	4	0	4
Hemoglobin	<11.0 g/dl	3	2	4	0	4
Serum Iron	<40 µg/dl	6	8	5	3	0
Serum Folate	<3 ng/dl	14	10	15	9	75
RBC Folate	<160 ng/dl	54	31	48	64	75
Serum Vitamin C	<0.2 mg/dl	2	5	0	2	4
Vitamin B$_6$	<1.8 units/dl	1	2	7	1	4
Serum Vitamin A	<20 µg/dl	14	2	0	3	0
Vitamin E	<700 µg/dl	22	36	61	26	25
Cholesterol	<250 mg/dl	1	0	4	6	5
Urinary Thiamine	<65 µg/gCr	3	4	0	5	0
Riboflavin	<79 µg/gCr	14	29	40	62	47
Niacin	<1.6 µg/gCr	3	2	0	3	0

from vending machine operations on their campuses, the financial implications cannot be overlooked.

Unless and until we can begin to answer and correct some of the above questions and problems, we can expect the adolescent female in the future to continue to enter her first pregnancy at significant nutritional risk before her reproductive effort ever begins.

REFERENCES

1. Committee on Adolescence, Group for the Advancement of Psychiatry: Normal Adolescence: Its Dynamics and Impact. New York, Charles Scribner's Sons, 1968
2. Heald FP (ed): Adolescent Gynecology. Baltimore, Williams & Wilkins, 1966
3. Heald FP, Daugela M, Brunschuyler P: Physiology of adolescence. N Engl J Med 268:192–198, 243–252, 299–307, 361–366, 1963
4. Huenemann RL, Shapiro LR, Hampton MC, Mitchell BW: Food and eating practices of teenagers. J Am Diet Assoc 53:17, 1968
5. Relation of nutrition to pregnancy in adolescence: a review. Clin Obstet Gynecol 14:367, 1971
6. Sabry ZI, Campbell JA, Campbell ME, Forbes AL: Nutrition Canada. Nutr Today 9:5, 1974
7. Salhanik HA, Kipins DM, Van de Wiele RL (eds): Metabolic Effects of Gonadal Hormones and Contraceptive Steroids. New York, Plenum Press, 1969
8. Tanner JM: The development of the female reproductive system during adolescence. Clin Obstet Gynecol 3:135, 1960
9. Tanner JM (ed): Growth at Adolescence, 2nd ed. Oxford, Blackwell, 1962
10. Theuer RC: Effect of oral contraceptive agents on vitamin and mineral needs: a review. J Reprod Med 8:13, 1972
11. Trowbridge FL, Hand KA, Nichaman MZ: Findings relating to goiter and iodine in the Ten State Nutrition Survey. Am J Clin Nutr 28:712, 1975
12. Trowbridge FL, Matovinovic J, McClaren G, Nichaman MZ: Iodine and goiter in children. Pediatrics 56:82, 1975
13. US Dept of Health, Education and Welfare. Nutrition evaluation of the population of Central America and Panama 1965–67. Washington DC, No. 72–8120, 1972
14. US Dept of Health, Education and Welfare. Ten State Nutrition Survey: 1968–1970. Washington DC, Publ No. 72–8131, 1972
15. WHO: Health problems of adolescence. (Tech Rep No. 308) Geneva, 1965
16. Young CM, Sipin SS, Roe DA: Body composition of preadolescent and adolescent girls. J Am Diet Assoc 53:25, 1968

Chapter 5

Effects of Maternal Dietary Restrictions During Pregnancy on Fetal Growth and Maternal-Fetal Exchange in the Mammalian Species

Pedro Rosso

The possibility that dietetic manipulation of any type may harm the fetus imposes methodologic problems and ethical considerations which make it extremely difficult to investigate the nutritional interactions between mother and fetus in human subjects. Therefore, the use of animal models is a major source of information. Experimental work with animals is performed under strictly controlled conditions, and maternal and fetal organs can be analyzed for histologic and biochemical changes. This approach has its shortcomings because of the significant differences that exist among mammalian species regarding certain important aspects of pregnancy such as rate of fetal growth, number of fetuses, or the proportion between maternal weight and weight of the conceptus at term. These differences limit the possibility of making extrapolations to humans or comparisons among species. However, eutherian mammals also share some important general characteristics. The most basic are a total dependency of the fetus on maternal supply, the increase in fetal requirements as pregnancy advances, and fetal growth retardation when the maternal diet is restricted during pregnancy. Because of these similarities, the study of maternal nutrition and fetal–maternal interaction in other species has become a source of valuable information providing a better interpretation of the human situation.

This chapter reviews the current information on the effects of maternal caloric or protein restriction during pregnancy on fetal growth. The effects of vitamin and mineral deficiencies on fetal growth have been the subject of recent publications (17,26). Since a great majority of the work regarding dietary restrictions on prenatal growth has been done in rats, the review will focus on this species.

CHARACTERISTICS AND MECHANISMS OF NORMAL FETAL GROWTH

For all mammals, fetal life begins as one cell, which multiplies itself several billion times before birth. The rate at which this multiplication proceeds determines the substantial variation in birth weight and mean daily increment in fetal body weight among the different species. For example, the mouse fetus grows at a rate of 0.090 g a day, whereas, the blue whale fetus grows at a rate of 9,000 g a day, a variation by a factor of 100,000. By contrast, the length of gestation in the mouse compared to the length of gestation in the blue whale varies by a factor of 15.7 (Table 5–1). Thus, interspecies differences in fetal size at birth are a function of the fetal growth rate and not the length of gestation.

Proliferative growth of the fetus has been monitored using DNA content of the whole body and of different organs as an index of cell number and the protein/DNA ratio as an index of cell size (13,50). Using this method to study the characteristics of prenatal and postnatal growth in the rat has shown that normal growth is a sequence of three consecutive, somewhat overlapping, phases (48). During the first phase, organs grow exclusively by increasing their cell number. This is reflected by linear increases in DNA content of organs without changes in the protein/DNA ratio. Therefore, while cells are multiplying they maintain a constant size. During the second phase, the rate of cell division falls, and cell size begins to increase. Finally, in the third phase, cells have ceased dividing, and both organ growth and total body growth become a function of the increase in cell size or protein/DNA ratios. These phases have been called hyperplastic or proliferative, intermediate, and hypertrophic, respectively.

In the rat (50), man (46), and probably most other mammalian species, prenatal growth is mainly proliferative. At birth the DNA content of various organs of the rat is still increasing linearly (Fig. 5–1). In most organs, these linear increments continue during the first month of life with the exception of lungs and brain, in which the proliferative phase of growth is completed by days 18 and 21 of age, respectively (13,50).

FETAL NUTRIENT REQUIREMENTS DURING GESTATION

The linear increment in cell number of different fetal organs causes a linear increase in body weight during the last part of gestation. Since the fetus needs nutrients for the synthesis of new cells and tissues, the linear increment in body weight can be considered the cause of the rise in nutrient requirements. Thus, in the rat, as in other species, the need for nutrients increases near term.

Between conception and birth the nutritional needs of the fetus are met by three different mechanisms (45). During the preimplantation phase (which varies among different species), the blastocyst presumably absorbs nutrients through its outer layer of cells, the trophoblast. From implantation until establishment of the placental circulation, a sinusoidal space is formed between the fetal and maternal side, and conceivably the embryo receives nutrients directly from the maternal blood. Finally, the placenta develops, and the fetus receives its nutrients via the placental circulation. Thus, the placenta has a central role in pregnancy. Its primary functions involve the transfer of nutrients to the fetus and the induction of certain metabolic changes in the maternal organism that are essential for fetal survival and well being.

Table 5–1. RATE OF GROWTH OF DIFFERENT MAMMALS BEFORE BIRTH.*

Species	Length of gestation (days)	Weight at birth (g)	Mean growth rate (g/day)
Mouse	21	2	0.09
Rat	21	5	0.24
Cat	63	100	1.6
Dog	63	200	3.2
Pig	120	1500	4.2
Man	280	3500	12.5
Elephant	600	114000	190
Hippopotamus	240	50000	210
Blue whale	330	3000000	9000

*Widdowson EM: Proc Nutr Soc 28:17, 1968

Fig. 5–1. DNA content in different organs and the whole animal during prenatal and postnatal growth of the rat. Values represent means and ranges for at least 10 animals or organs. (Winick M; Noble A: Dev Biol 12:451, 1965)

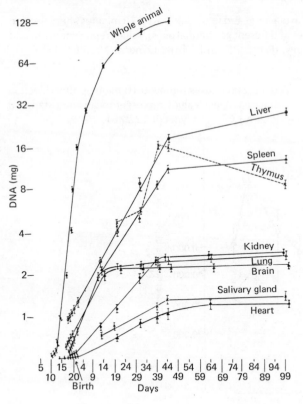

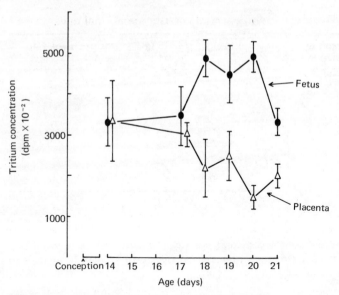

Fig. 5–2. Concentration of tritium in placenta and fetuses removed 10 minutes after injection of D-glucose-1-(^{3}H) into the mother at different gestational ages. Values represent mean and standard error of three to six values. (Rosso P: Am J Obstet Gynecol 122:761, 1975)

Fig. 5–3. Concentration of AIB in placentas and fetuses removed 10 minutes after injection of AIB into the mother at different gestational ages. Values represent means and standard error of four to five samples. (Rosso P: Am J Obstet Gynecol 122:761, 1975)

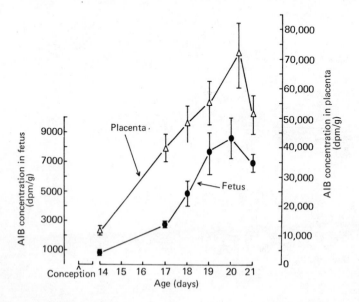

The basic nutritional needs of the fetus at different gestational ages are unknown. Traditionally, glucose was believed to supply all of the substrate required for fetal oxidative metabolism in most mammalian species. However, recent evidence indicates that in fetal lambs near term, amino acid catabolism supplies a considerable amount of substrate for aerobic metabolism (43).

Thus, the adequate transfer of glucose and amino acids into the fetus is essential for normal fetal growth. Recent experiments with rats have demonstrated that during the last week of gestation there is a substantial increase in the capacity of the placenta to transfer glucose and α-amino isobutyric acid (AIB), a nonmetabolizable amino acid (32). In these studies, labeled glucose and AIB were injected into the maternal circulation, and the concentration of label measured in placenta and fetuses removed at different time intervals. The data demonstrates that between days 14 and 20 of gestation there is a progressive tenfold increase in the concentration of AIB. By contrast, the concentration of glucose increases only after day 17 of gestation (Fig. 5–2 and 5–3).

A parallel increase in the concentration of AIB in the placental and fetal tissues reflects an increased placental capacity to take up and concentrate this substance. This is reflected by the rate of transfer of AIB and glucose per gram of placental tissue per unit of time. Between day 14 and day 21 of gestation, the rate increases approximately 100 times for AIB and proportionally less for glucose. Therefore, the increased transfer of nutrients does not seem to be solely a function of increasing fetal size but rather of an increased ability of the placenta to take up nutrients from the maternal circulation and then transfer them into the fetus. These changes reflect a previously unknown phenomenon of placental maturation.

Table 5–2. WEIGHTS OF MOTHERS AND YOUNG, AND LENGTHS OF GESTATION IN MAN AND SOME COMMON LABORATORY SPECIES*

Species	Maternal weight (kg)	Birth weight (gm)	Birth weight in terms of maternal weight (%)		Usual number of young
			Single fetus	Whole litter	
Man	56	3200	5.7	5.7	1
Pig	130	1200	1.1	6.8	8
Sheep (Hampshire)	70	4000	5.7	11.4	2
Dog (beagle)	8.4	270	3.2	16.1	5
Rhesus monkey	8	500	6.3	6.3	1
Cat	3	100	3.3	13.2	4
Rabbit	2.5	50	2.0	14.0	7
Guinea pig	0.7	85	12.1	36.3	3
Rat	0.15	5	3.3	23.4	7
Mouse	0.03	1.4	4.7	37.3	8

*Dawes GS: Fetal and Neonatal Physiology: a comparative study of the changes at birth. Chicago, Year Book Medical, 1969

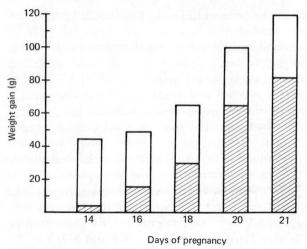

Fig. 5–4. Maternal weight *(open columns)* and conceptus weight gain *(hatched columns)* during the last week of pregnancy in the rat. Values represent mean differences over nonpregnant rats of similar size and age. A total of 8 rats were used in each group. (Rosso P: unpublished observations)

Fig. 5–5. Changes in the composition of the maternal carcass (moisture, *hatched columns;* protein, *open columns;* fat, *solid columns*) during the last week of gestation. (Beaton GH, Beare J, Ryu MH, McHenry EW: J Nutr 54:291, 1954)

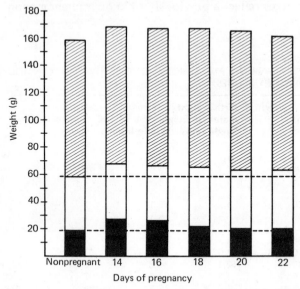

MATERNAL ADAPTATIONS TO PREGNANCY

The nutritional needs of the conceptus determine a nutritional stress in the mother that is highest in multiparous mammals. In small rodents, such as the rat or guinea pig, the weight of the conceptus at term may represent 25 or 37% of the maternal weight, respectively (12) (Table 5–2).

To meet the higher requirements of pregnancy, the maternal organism undergoes several adaptive changes such as increased food intake and deposition of body lipid and protein.

Increases in maternal food intake are evident usually at the end of the first third of pregnancy in the rat and other animals. The increase rises steadily, reaching a maximum near term (6). Parallel to this increased nutrient intake is a significant increase in body weight. Analysis of the maternal and fetal components of body weight at term shows that, besides the increase in conceptus weight, the mother has also gained weight significantly (Fig. 5–4).

Studies of body composition in the rat demonstrate that maternal weight gain during pregnancy reflects deposition of both protein and lipid on the maternal carcass (5). The laying down of these substances follows a certain sequence. Until day 16 of gestation a larger proportion of lipid than protein is deposited; after day 16 the situation is reversed (Fig. 5–5).

Balance studies demonstrate that nitrogen deposition in the maternal carcass begins after the first week of pregnancy. By day 14 of gestation, only 17.6% of the additional 748.6 mg of nitrogen retained in pregnant animals is present in the conceptus. The rest is distributed in muscle, liver, and other organs of the mother. The situation is considerably reversed at day 21. Only 15.7% of the total nitrogen retention over nonpregnant levels (220.7 mg) is in maternal stores and the rest is in the conceptus (24). This shift has been interpreted as indicating an initial anabolic phase up to 14 days followed by a catabolic phase in which amino acid from maternal protein are transported into the fetus.

The higher nitrogen retention reflects greater availability of amino acids secondary to increased maternal intake. This also reflects a net increase in nitrogen retention. This effect is attained by reducing both urea synthesis and the activity of liver enzymes such as alanine aminotransferase and alanineglutamic transaminase (5,24). By day 21 of pregnancy, these hepatic changes produce an effect that spares amino acid which represents an additional amount of nitrogen retained equivalent to 45% of the total nitrogen products accumulated in the conceptus (25).

EFFECTS OF MATERNAL DIETARY RESTRICTION DURING PREGNANCY ON FETAL GROWTH

Reduced caloric or protein intake during pregnancy causes reduced birth weight in several mammalian species, including man. Nearly 30 years ago, the phenomenon was investigated in sheep (44). A group of sheep were underfed 28 to day 91 of pregnancy (length of gestation in sheep is 147 days)

quently overfed until delivery. Another group was treated in the reverse order. It was found that maternal dietary restriction during the last 60 days of pregnancy caused an approximate 40% reduction in birth weight. No effect on birth weight was observed in the underfed–overfed group. The data also showed marked metabolic changes in the underfed ewes during the last part of pregnancy. Fatty liver and general somatic disturbances described as toxemia of pregnancy, including convulsions, were described. This condition is similar to human toxemia of pregnancy but without maternal hypertension. The fact that dietary restriction in sheep induces marked metabolic abnormalities suggests the possibility that other factors besides nutrition, such as vascular or hormonal changes, could have a negative influence on fetal growth.

In the rat, either a 50% overall reduction of food intake or a decrease in protein content of the diet, to 5–6%, throughout pregnancy caused a 25–30% lower birth weight (6, 9, 47, 55). More moderate restrictions of dietary protein caused a graded effect (25).

The decreased body weight of the neonates reflects a reduction in the weight of every organ measured (brain, liver, kidney, spleen, thymus, and intestines) (22, 47, 55, 59) (Table 5–3). Although the organ weight reduction is proportional to the reduction of body weight, some organs such as brain tend to be proportionally less affected (47) (Table 5–3). Most studies show that brain weight in pups from restricted mothers is only 15–23% less than in control animals (47, 54). By contrast, kidney, spleen, and thymus weights each tend to be proportionally more reduced than the body weight (22, 56).

Again in the rat, lower birth weight reflects a reduced rate of fetal growth during the last week of pregnancy. Before day 14 of pregnancy there are no significant differences between pups from control and restricted mothers. However, the trend toward smaller fetal size becomes noticeable in the restricted animals at day 16 of gestation, and the differences between the two groups are usually significant by day 20 or 21 of gestation (29).

Since prenatal growth is proliferative, the fetal growth retardation caused by maternal restriction of either calories or protein implies a reduced cell number in every organ. This fact is reflected by a lower DNA content of the pup's organs.

DNA content of the brain in the newborns of restricted mothers has been found to be reduced 10–15% when compared to newborns in a control group whose dames were fed 24% or 25% protein diets (47, 54).

Table 5–3. EFFECT OF MATERNAL MALNUTRITION ON FETAL TISSUES*

Tissue	Weight	Percent normal control Protein	RNA	DNA
Whole animal	87	81	83	81
Brain	91	85	82	84
Heart	84	84	79	81
Lung	82	85	85	89
Liver	82	80	85	85
Kidney	84	81	82	85

*Winick M: Cellular growth of the placenta as an indicator of abnormal fetal growth. In Adamson K (ed): Diagnosis and Treatment of Fetal Disorders. New York, Springer-Verlag, 1969

Reduced DNA content of the brain has been the focus of a considerable number of studies. The use of autoradiographic methods has determined that, by 16 days of age, fetuses from protein-restricted mothers have an overall reduction in the rate of cell division in the brain (53). This has been shown to follow a well-defined regional pattern determined by the rate of cell division in different areas of the brain. For example, in areas where at day 16 of gestation the rate of cell division is comparatively slow, such as the cerebral white and gray matter, the number of cells that incorporated labeled thymidine was moderately reduced when compared with that of control fetuses. Areas adjacent to the third ventricle and subiculum, where proportionally more cells are dividing at this age, were found to be proportionally more affected. Finally, the cerebellum and the area adjacent to the lateral ventricle had the most marked reduction in the number of dividing cells when compared to control samples (Fig. 5–6). These data indicate that the brain is not uniformly affected and that those areas more susceptible to the effects of prenatal nutrient deprivation are those with a higher rate of cell division.

A similar phenomenon has been described in rats suffering postnatal malnutrition from birth until 21 days of age. Increasing the size of the litter to 18 pups resulted in animals that were malnourished from birth. They were compared to animals reared in litters of 8. By 8 days of age the malnourished animals showed a reduced DNA content in cerebellum. When the animals were 14 days old, a lower DNA content of the cerebrum was demonstrated. At 21 days, comparison with control animals showed that the DNA content of cerebrum and cerebellum was reduced 25% and 35%, respectively (Fig. 5–7) (14). Studies on the normal growth of rat brain have shown that between birth and 21 days of age, increments in DNA content of the cerebellum are higher than in cerebrum, indicating that cerebellum has a faster proliferative growth (15). Thus, both prenatal and postnatal studies indicate that a reduced supply of nutrients interferes with the rate of cell division in the various organs and that the effect is proportionally more deleterious in tissues with a faster rate of cell division.

Studies conducted in rats malnourished from birth until 21 days of age have shown that the reduced DNA content of the various organs cannot be reversed by feeding the animals a normal diet *ad libitum* (51). These animals will remain smaller and will have fewer cells in the brain and other organs for the rest of their lives. The cause of this effect is still unknown. Apparently, the proliferative phase of growth is controlled by a precise biologic timer that turns off at a certain developmental stage regardless of the cellular events that may have occurred during this period. Therefore, from the point of view of ultimate growth achievements, the hyperplastic phase is a critical period.

Overfeeding rats during the hyperplastic phase of growth causes acceleration of the rate of cell division, producing a higher DNA content per organ (52). The model for these studies has been to raise animals in litters of 3 or 4 pups. By the end of the lactation period (21 days of age), these animals have an increased body size and increased DNA content in every organ, when compared to animals raised in litters of 8–10 pups.

Overfeeding during proliferative growth has been used to rehabilitate mal-

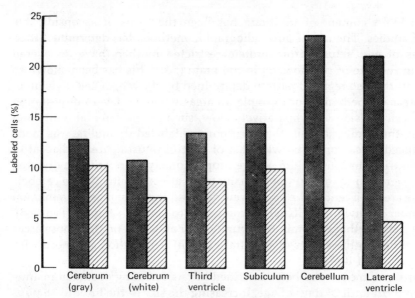

Fig. 5–6. Effect of maternal protein restriction *(hatched columns) compared to normal controls (shaded columns)* during pregnancy on various brain regions in 16-day fetus. (Winick M, Brasel JA, Rosso P: Nutrition and cell growth. In Winick M (ed): Current Concepts in Nutrition, I. New York, John Wiley, 1972)

Fig. 5–7. Effect of malnutrition from birth on DNA content of various regions of rat brain at different days. (Fish I, Winick M: Exp Neurol 25:534, 1969)

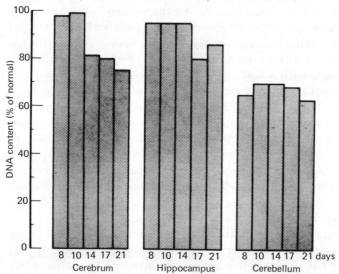

nourished pups when cell division is still occurring. By increasing litter size to 18 pups, pups have been malnourished from birth to 9 days of age, then nursed in litters of 4 until day 21. DNA content in the organs of these animals was found to be similar to control pups (49). Thus, permanent stunting caused by early malnutrition can be prevented with adequate rehabilitation if begun while cell division is still occurring.

Applying the principles just discussed to the prenatal situation, it seemed possible that overfeeding from birth could reverse the effects of maternal malnutrition. As previously mentioned, the only organs in which cell proliferation ends before weaning are lungs and brain. In those organs the deficit in DNA content is relatively small, and so it appears easily correctable within this 3-week time limit. However, the problem of recovering from a prenatal deficit in cell number appears to be considerably more complex than predicted.

The brain is made up of an heterogenous cell population that broadly can be categorized as belonging to two basic groups—neurons and glial cells. Each type of cell has its own unique timing for proliferative growth. In the rat, neurons demonstrate proliferative growth, almost exclusively during prenatal life (4). By contrast, the bulk of glial cells is still actively dividing for some time after birth. DNA polymerase studies in the rat indicate that the peak of glial cell division occurs at day 10 of postnatal life (7). Therefore, it is conceivable that the 10–15% reduction in brain DNA content at birth caused by maternal protein malnutrition represents a reduction in neuronal cells. Since at birth these cells have already ceased to divide, they would not be affected by any dietary rehabilitation. Furthermore, postnatal nutritional recovery is likely to accelerate proliferative growth of glial cells. Histologic studies done in progeny of protein-restricted rats support this hypothesis by demonstrating a larger proportion of glial cells during postnatal recovery (36).

The effect of maternal deprivation on organs other than brain is still relatively unexplored. It has been demonstrated that thymus and spleen are among the organs most affected by maternal restriction, and as previously mentioned, the weight of these organs at birth frequently is proportionally more reduced than body weight in the malnourished pups (22). More detailed studies have been done with kidney. Progeny of rats fed a 6% casein diet throughout pregnancy have smaller kidneys, with a reduction in less differentiated glomeruli and with fewer collecting ducts. Proximal tubules are also shorter and less convoluted (1, 56). At 6 days of age these pups have a reduced response to either water or osmotic diuresis when compared to the progeny of rats fed a 24% casein diet (18). When tested at day 22, these pups were also found to have a reduced rate of glomerular filtration (3).

Histologic and functional changes in the intestines of the prenatally malnourished rats have also been reported (23). Smaller diameter and shortening of the jejunal villi, with histologic evidence of a decreased absorption of protein and fat by jejunal enterocytes, were the main changes reported. In addition, cells in which the absorptive defect was most evident had a decreased content of cytoplasmic organelles. Opposite findings have been described in guinea pigs born from protein-deficient mothers (60).

LASTING EFFECTS OF MATERNAL MALNUTRITION DURING PREGNANCY

Progeny of mothers fed either a low-protein or a calorie-restricted diet, or both, remain smaller throughout life (11, 58). However, when adults the deficit in body weight is smaller than found at birth (Fig. 5–8). Studies show the deficit in body weight to be approximately 20% at 21 days of age (57), 12% at 76 days of age (8), and only 8–10% in older males (10). The reduced body size seems to reflect shortening of the long bones (1). Studies on skeletal development demonstrate that these animals have retarded ossification which is apparent at day 17 of gestation. At this age the retarded ossification was estimated to be a developmental lag of 24 hours. The difference became more evident postnatally, with a 4-day lag in bone center development during the first weeks of life (34).

The rate of bone elongation is also significantly slower in the progeny from dams fed a protein-restricted diet. At 65 and 90 days of age, tibial elongation per day is similar in control and prenatally restricted animals, while body weight is increasing proportionally faster in the deficient rats, suggesting that bone growth may be affected specifically (34).

In the study of the possible lasting consequences of prenatal malnutrition, the area that has attracted most attention is the possible functional consequences of a reduced brain DNA content. The model used in these studies has also been maternal protein restriction during gestation, with subsequent adjustment of litter size to 4 or 8–10 pups and refeeding of the mother with an adequate protein diet or using of an adequately nourished foster mother from birth.

Animals from protein-restricted mothers reared in litters of 4 pups have

Fig. 5–8. Changes in postnatal body weight in progeny from diet-restricted mother (50% of control intake) and control rats. (Chow BF, Rider AA: J Anim Sci 36:167, 1973)

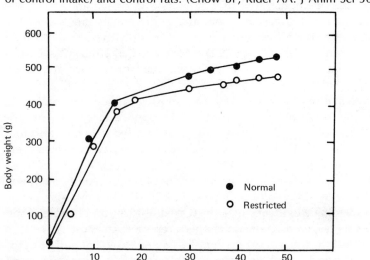

reduced DNA content of the brain at 21 days of age (57). Since no further cell division is expected to occur in brain after this age, one would predict a lasting deficit in brain DNA. However, no differences in DNA content of the brain between controls and the progeny of restricted mothers has been found in 6-month-old animals (41). Studies on functional aspects of the brain have shown that the progeny of protein-restricted mothers have a series of behavioral changes and learning incompetence when they become adults. Behavioral and emotional responses have been measured by observing the performance of these animals in an open field and their interactions with the other animals or by introducing abnormal stimuli such as electric shock. These observations demonstrate that animals from protein-restricted mothers have a tendency to take bizarre stances and, in general, show an increased liability to disruption of behavior when they become adults (20, 35, 39, 40). Furthermore, their interaction with other animals demonstrates that they have "antigroup" attitudes with fluctuating dominant–submissive behavior (11) (Fig. 5–9).

Prenatally undernourished animals also seem to have a reduced capacity to learn when confronted with tests such as the T maze, the Lahsley III water maze, and the pole-jump avoidance test (8, 37).

Comparisons between progeny of mothers with protein-restricted diets and

Fig. 5–9. Number of licks to a water receptacle made by control rats *(solid line)* and progeny of rats malnourished during pregnancy *(dashed line)* before *(BS)* and after *(AS)* receiving an electric shock from the receptacle. Values represent number of licks at different trials during a 60-second period following the first lick. (Hanson HM, Simonson M: Nutr Rep Int 4:307, 1971)

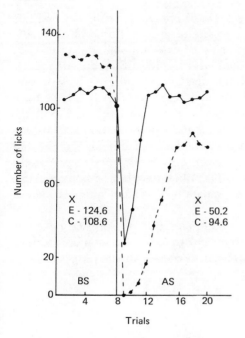

mothers with calorie-restricted diets indicate that the lasting behavioral abnormalities are associated exclusively with protein deficiency. Since the effects of both types of restrictions are similar on birth weight and, conceivably, on the weight of other organs, the data suggest a specific effect on brain caused by the reduced availability of amino acids secondary to the protein-restricted diet (27, 28).

Long-lasting changes have also been reported on kidneys. Pups from restricted mothers were reared in litters of 4 animals, a situation that, as previously discussed, causes accelerated growth. Although there was a partial recovery in DNA content of the kidneys in these animals, the cellularity is restricted to existing nephrons and to a lengthening of the proximal convoluted tubes (2). Thus, prenatal growth retardation due to maternal malnutrition seems to cause a permanent abnormality of the structure and functional capacity of the kidneys.

Considering their slightly reduced DNA content, lungs seem to be the organ least affected by prenatal deficiency in the rat (47). However, there is evidence that lung metabolism is significantly altered (21). Progeny of rats fed a 10% casein diet throughout pregnancy were compared with those of a control group fed a 27% casein diet. At birth the respiratory control index of mitochondria from deficient rats was significantly reduced. A similar reduction was also found in the amount of ADP utilized. This would be indirect evidence of a reduced rate of ATP synthesis in the lungs.

In contrast, spleen and thymus are able to attain a weight similar to control animals within a few days. No abnormalities have been found in the capacity of the prenatally malnourished rat to develop a normal immune response later in life (22).

There is evidence that the endocrine system of prenatally malnourished rats may also be altered. Comparing the *in vitro* rate of growth hormone synthesis and release in pituitaries of 36-day-old male control animals and prenatally restricted animals shows that these functions were significantly reduced in pituitaries of deficient animals (35). Lower plasma levels and pituitary concentration of growth hormone in progeny of rats fed a 50% restricted diet (42) have been reported.

Further support of the possibility that altered endocrine function may be one of the mechanisms by which postnatal recovery of deficient animals is prevented is given by data showing that administration of growth hormone to prenatally malnourished pups increases epiphyseal width, tibial length, and body weight. These findings suggest that bones from prenatally restricted animals have a normal growth potential (58).

Moreover, it has also been reported that administration of a pituitary extract, and to a lesser extent growth hormone, from day 7 to 28 of postnatal life reduced considerably behavioral abnormalities present in these animals (38).

MATERNAL–FETAL INTERACTIONS DURING DIETARY RESTRICTIONS

It has been postulated that nutrients are distributed from the maternal blood into the various tissues according to metabolic needs; thus, tissues that are more active metabolically receive a greater proportion of materials (19). During pregnancy the conceptus participates in this partition and, based on its higher metabolic rate, would receive more nutrients per unit weight than the mother.

If nutrients become less available, the fetus would compete advantageously with the maternal organs. As the limitation becomes more severe the fetus would receive a proportionally larger share of nutrients (16).

Evidence that fetal growth is affected only when the restriction of calories and/or protein during pregnancy are extreme seem to support the *fetal parasitism* hypothesis. However, there are several facts that are difficult to explain by this hypothesis.

When changes in maternal body weight in a group of rats fed either a 6% or a 27% casein diet (from day 5 of gestation) are analyzed at term after removal of the uterus and the conceptus, rats fed a 27% casein diet weigh more. However, when these weights are compared to nonpregnant female rats of similar age and size fed similar diets for the same length of time, it is evident that while the control pregnant group has gained additional weight, the protein-restricted rats have not lost a significant amount of weight (Fig. 5–10).

A similar correlation has been found when rats from a 50% overall restricted diet were compared with nonrestricted pregnant and restricted and unrestricted nonpregnant females (6, 10). Results suggest that, under conditions of severe protein or dietary restrictions imposed during pregnancy, the mother does not use a significant amount of her own tissue to support fetal growth. Further, the comparison of percent loss of body weight in mother and conceptus in rats fed a 6% casein diet demonstrate that the conceptus is affected proportionally more than the mother (Fig. 5–11). Thus, the capacity of the fetus to compete for available nutrients and to parasitize the mother does not seem to be as effective as postulated. Further, fetal parasitism seems to be limited mainly to utilization of those nutrients normally deposited in maternal stores by the mother.

The mother can limit the transfer of nutrients into the fetus either by increasing its metabolic rate, by decreasing the metabolic rate of the fetus, or by reducing the rate of transfer of nutrients into the fetus.

Recent data indicate that the latter mechanism is used by rats fed a 6% casein diet during pregnancy. It was found that after injecting either labeled glucose or AIB into the maternal circulation, the concentration of label found in placenta and fetuses 10 minutes later was lower in protein-restricted animals than in controls (30, 31) (Fig. 5–12). The characteristics of the phenomenon have not been yet defined. The most likely possibilities are that either the maternal blood perfusion to the pregnant uterus or the capacity of the placenta to transfer nutrients or both are decreased.

Indirect evidence that placental transfer of AIB could be impaired shows a proportionally higher concentration of AIB in the placenta than the fetus in the

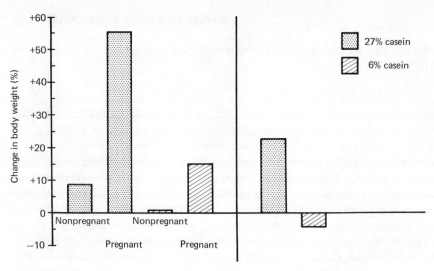

Fig. 5–10. Changes in maternal body weight (A) at day 21 in pregnant and nonpregnant rats fed a 6% *(Hatched columns)* or a 27% *(dotted columns)* casein diet from day 6 of pregnancy. (B) Changes in maternal body weight at day 21 after removal of the conceptus in pregnant rats fed a 6% *(Hatched columns)* or a 27% *(dotted columns)* casein diet from day 6 of pregnancy. Values represent mean of 8 animals in each group. (Rosso P, Wasserman M: Unpublished observations)

Fig. 5–11. Percent reduction in maternal weight (after removal of the conceptus) and weight of the conceptus in rats fed a 6% casein diet from day 6 of gestation. Weight of the conceptus is compared with weight of conceptus from rats fed a 27% diet during pregnancy. Maternal weight is compared with weight of nonpregnant rats of similar size and age fed a 6% casein diet. Values represent means from 8 animals and 8 litters. (Rosso P: Unpublished observations)

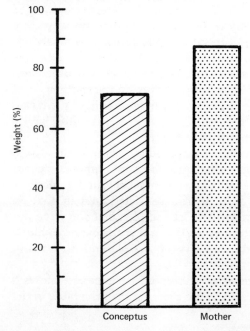

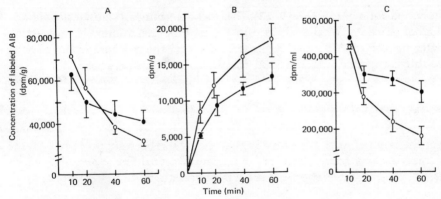

Fig. 5–12. Concentration of ^{14}C-labeled AIB expressed as disintegrations per minute per gram or per milliliter in placenta (A), fetuses (B), and maternal plasma (C) of rats fed a 27% *(open circles)* or 6% *(solid circles)* casein diet at different times after intravenous administration of the label to the mother. (Rosso P: Science 187:648, 1975. Copyright 1975 by the American Association for the Advancement of Science.)

Fig. 5–13. The ratio of AIB concentration in the fetus to that in the placenta in normal *(open columns)* and malnourished *(hatched columns)* rats at various times after intravenous injection of AIB into the maternal circulation. (Rosso P: Science 187:648, 1975. Copyright 1975 by the American Association for the Advancement of Science.)

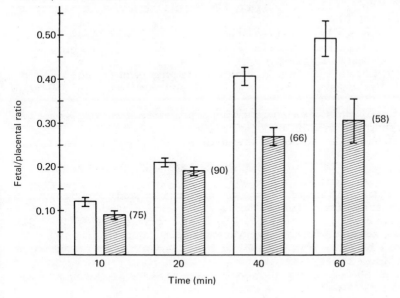

malnourished animals (31) (Fig. 5–13). This fact determines a statistically significant higher placental/fetal AIB ratio in the malnourished animals, suggesting that after uptake of AIB from the maternal blood the placenta is not able to release this compound into the fetal circulation at a normal speed.

ACKNOWLEDGMENTS

Some of the original work presented in this review has been supported by grants from The Nutrition Foundation, 487-F.L., The National Foundation-March of Dimes, 1–285, and the National Institutes of Health, 5-R22 H D 06682.

REFERENCES

1. Allen LH, Zeman FJ: Influence of increased postnatal food intake on body composition of progeny of protein-deficient rats. J Nutr 101: 1311, 1971
2. Allen LH, Zeman FJ: Influence of increased postnatal nutrient intake on kidney cellular development in progeny of protein-deficient rats. J Nutr 103:929 1973
3. Allen LH, Zeman FJ: Kidney function in the progeny of protein-deficient rats. J Nutr 103: 1467, 1973
4. Altman J, Das GD: Autoradiographic and histological studies of postnatal neurogenesis. J Comp Neurol 126:337, 1966
5. Beaton GH, Beare J, Ryu MH, McHenry EW: Protein metabolism in the pregnant rat. J Nutr 54:291, 1954
6. Berg BN: Dietary restriction and reproduction in the rat. J Nutr 87:344, 1965
7. Brasel JA, Ehrenkranz RA, Winick M: DNA polymerase activity in rat brain during ontogeny. Dev Biol 23:424, 1970
8. Caldwell DF, Churchill JA: Learning ability in the progeny of rats administered a protein-deficient diet during the second half of gestation. Neurology (Minneap) 17:95, 1967
9. Chow BF, Lee CJ: Effect of dietary restriction of pregnant rats on body weight gain of the offspring. J Nutr 82:10, 1964
10. Chow BF, Rider AA: Implications of the effects of maternal diet in various species. J Anim Sci 36:167, 1973
11. Chow BF, Simonson M, Hanson HM, Roeder LM: Behavioral measurements in nutritional studies. Cond Reflex 6:36, 1971
12. Dawes GS: Fetal and Neonatal Physiology: a comparative study of the changes at birth. Chicago, Year Book Medical, 1969
13. Enesco L, Leblond CP: Increase in cell number as a factor in the growth of the organs of the young male rat. J Embryol Exp Morphol 10:530, 1962
14. Fish I, Winick M: Effect of malnutrition on regional growth of the developing rat brain. Exp Neurol 25:534, 1969
15. Fish I, Winick M: Cellular growth in various regions of the developing rat brain. Pediatr Res 3:407, 1969
16. Frazer JFD, Huggett AS: The partition of nutrients between mother and conceptus in the pregnant rat. J Physiol (Lond) 207:783, 1970
17. Giroud A: Nutrition of the embryo. Fed Proc 27:163, 1968
18. Hall SM, Zeman FJ: Kidney function of the progeny of rats fed a low protein diet. J Nutr 95:49, 1968
19. Hammond J: Physiological factors affecting birth weight. Proc Nutr Soc 2:8, 1944
20. Hanson HM, Simonson M: Effects of fetal undernourishment on experimental anxiety. Nutr Rep Int 4:307, 1971

21. Hawrylewicz EJ, Kissane JQ, Blair WH, Heppner CA: Effect of maternal protein malnutrition on neonatal lung development and mitochondrial function. Nutr Rep Int 7:253, 1973.

22. Kenney MA: Development of spleen and thymus in offspring of protein-deficient rats. J Nutr 98:202, 1969

23. Loh K–R W, Shrader RE, Zeman FJ: Effect of maternal protein deprivation on neonatal intestinal absorption in rats. J Nutr 101:1663, 1971

24. Naismith DJ: The fetus as a parasite. Proc Nutr Soc 28:25, 1969

25. Naismith DJ: Adaptations in the metabolism of protein during pregnancy and their nutritional implications. Nutr Rep Int 7:383, 1973

26. Prasad A, Oberleas D: Trace elements in maternal and fetal nutrition. In Moghissi KS (ed): Birth Defects and Fetal Development. Springfield, Ill, CC Thomas, 1974

27. Rider AA, Simonson M: Effect on rat offspring of maternal diet deficient in calories but not in protein. Nutr Rep Int 7:361, 1973

28. Rider AA, Simonson M: The relationship between maternal diet, birth weight and behavior of the offspring in the rat. Nutr Rep Int 10:19, 1974

29. Rosso P: Unpublished observations

30. Rosso P: Maternal malnutrition and placental transfer of nutrients in the rat (abstr). Pediatr Res 8:359, 1974

31. Rosso P: Maternal malnutrition and placental transfer of α-amino isobutyric acid in the rat. Science 187:648, 1975

32. Rosso P: Changes in the transfer of nutrients across the placenta during normal gestation in the rat. Am J Obstet Gynecol 122:761, 1975

33. Rosso P, Wasserman M: Unpublished observations

34. Shrader RE, Zeman FJ: Skeletal development in rats as affected by maternal protein deprivation and postnatal food supply. J Nutr 193:792, 1973

35. Shrader RE, Zeman FJ: In vitro synthesis of anterior pituitary growth hormone as affected by maternal protein deprivation and postnatal food supply. J Nutr 103:1012, 1973

36. Siassi F, Siassi B: Differential effects of protein-calorie restriction and subsequent repletion in neuronal and nonneuronal components of cerebral cortex in newborn rats. J Nutr 103:1625, 1973

37. Simonson M, Chow FB: Maze studies on progeny of underfed mother rats. J Nutr 101: 331, 1971

38. Simonson M, Hanson HM, Roeder LM, Chow BF: Effects of growth hormone and pituitary extract on behavioral abnormalities in offspring of undernourished rats. Nutr Rep Int 7:321, 1973

39. Simonson M, Sherwin RW, Anilane JK, Yu WY, Chow BF: Neuromotor development in progeny of underfed mother rats. J Nutr 98:18, 1969

40. Simonson M, Stephan JK, Hanson HM, Chow BF: Open field studies in offspring of underfed mother rats. J Nutr 101:331, 1971

41. Stephan JK: The permanent effect of prenatal dietary restriction on the brain of the progeny. Nutr Rep Int 4:257, 1971

42. Stephan JK, Vhow B, Frohman LA, Chow BF: Relationship of growth hormone to the growth retardation associated with maternal dietary restriction. J Nutr 101:1453, 1971

43. Tsoulos NG, Colwill JR, Battaglia FC, Makowski EL, Meschia G: Comparison of glucose, fructose and O^2 uptakes by the fetuses of fed and starved ewes. Am J Physiol 221:234, 1971

44. Wallace LR: The effect of diet on foetal development (abstr). J Physiol (Lond) 104:34–35P, 1945

45. Widdowson EM: How the foetus is fed. Proc Nutr Soc 28:17, 1968

46. Widdowson EM, Crabb DE, Milner RDG: Cellular development of some human organs before birth. Arch Dis Child 47:652, 1972

47. Winick M: Cellular growth of the placenta as an indicator of abnormal fetal growth.

In Adamson K (ed): Diagnosis and Treatment of Fetal Disorders. New York, Springer–Verlag, 1969, pp 83–101

48. Winick M, Brasel JA, Rosso P: Nutrition and cell growth. In Winick M (ed): Current Concepts in Nutrition, I. New York, John Wiley, 1972

49. Winick M, Fish I, Rosso P: Cellular recovery in rat tissues after a brief period of neonatal malnutrition. J Nutr 95:623, 1968

50. Winick M, Noble A: Quantitative changes in DNA, RNA and protein during prenatal and postnatal growth in the rat. Dev Biol 12:451, 1965

51. Winick M, Noble A: Cellular response in rats during malnutrition at various ages. J Nutr 89:300, 1966

52. Winick M, Noble A: Cellular response with increased feeding in neonatal rats. J Nutr 91:179, 1967

53. Winick M, Rosso P: Malnutrition and central nervous system development. In Prescott JW, Read M, Coursin D (eds): Brain Function and Malnutrition: Neuropsychological Methods of Assessment. New York, John Wiley, 1975, p 41

54. Zamenhoff S, Van Marthens E, Margolis FL: DNA (cell number) and protein in neonatal brain: alteration by maternal dietary protein restriction. Science 160:322, 1968

55. Zeman FJ: Effect on the young rat of maternal protein restriction. J Nutr 93: 167, 1967

56. Zeman FJ: Effects of maternal protein restriction on the kidney of the newborn young of rats. J Nutr 94:111, 1968

57. Zeman FJ: Effect of protein deficiency during gestation on postnatal cellular development in the young rat. J Nutr 100:530, 1970

58. Zeman FJ, Shrader RE, Allen LH: Persistent effects of maternal protein deficiency in postnatal rats. Nutr Rep Int 7:421, 1973

59. Zeman FJ, Stanbrough EC: Effect of maternal protein deficiency on cellular development in the fetal rat. J Nutr 99:274, 1969

60. Zeman FJ, Widdowson EM: Lipid absorption in newborn young of guinea pigs fed a protein-deficient diet during gestation. Biol Neonate 24:344, 1974

Chapter 6

Factors in Intrauterine Impoverishment

John A. Churchill

Medical thought has traditionally considered any baby weighing 2.5 kg to be premature. Unlike the well-known high mortality risk in small babies, the matter of neurologic morbidity in such low-birth-weight infants has been little understood. Until recently, medical opinion remained essentially unchanged since the literature of a century ago cited prematurity, along with other obstetric difficulties, as the cause of all forms of congenital neurologic defects including mental retardation and cerebral palsy (15). Only within the last few years has the medical world recognized that all low-birth-weight infants are not premature and that the fate of small full-term infants differs significantly from that of premature infants.

Children with spastic diplegia cerebral palsy were found to be almost always born prematurely, while children with mental retardation were rarely premature (5). Conversely, the mentally retarded were born small but at term (2). Despite contrary opinions, Alm's study of prematurity supported this conclusion by revealing no increase in mental retardation in premature infants (1). His measure of prematurity was gestational age, not birth weight. Likewise, Macdonald found no mental retardation in premature infants after discounting those with cerebral palsy (16).

In a previously published study, we examined the association of IQ and birth weight with bright school children contrasted to retarded school children (10). The results showed that birth weight—not duration of pregnancy—is the important factor. Later, we designed a study using identical twins which proved that IQ varied with birth weight independently of gestational age (21).

From this study, we determined that some babies are stunted *in utero,* with a blighting effect being exerted on brain as well as on other body structures. The general absence of malformations and lack of evidence of genetic, infectious, and other obvious factors suggested that the commonest causes might be found in either the incapability of the mother to supply nutrients to the fetus or the inability of the fetal placenta to extract sustenance from the mother. The term *intrauterine impoverishment* was coined to describe the theory.

To illustrate the problem of intrauterine impoverishment and its relationship to both birth weight and mental capability, a simple study using clinical case data was prepared. The study included the first 50 consecutive cases of learning disability in my data file. Those subjects having multiple malformations or specific nosologic disease entities were excluded. The cases were thus all in the large category of undifferentiated mental subnormality or learning disability.

In this study, the controls used were siblings of the subjects, so that the subject could not have been an only child and the birth weight of the sibling had to have been known. In any case with several siblings, only the one closest to the subject in age was made the control. Subjects with gestational ages equal to or greater than 38 weeks were included. No attempt was made to adjust the small differences in birth weight attributed to sex or parity. Male subjects exceed male controls in number; little difference in parity was seen. Various factors of maternal health were also tabulated.

Table 6–1 shows a clear difference in birth weight between subjects with learning disability and their sibling controls. In only five instances did the subject exceed his or her sibling's weight. It is noteworthy that many of the subjects with learning disability had birth weights well within the normal range but, nevertheless, were much smaller than their siblings.

POSSIBLE FACTORS CAUSING INTRAUTERINE IMPOVERISHMENT

Table 6–2 shows factors present during pregnancy which could have been responsible for intrauterine impoverishment. The factors are included to present ideas, but as derived, these data do not provide a basis to show statistical associations. In discussing these factors, other studies will be referred to for documentation of the role of the variables.

Table 6–1. COMPARISON OF SUBJECTS WITH LEARNING DISABILITIES AND THEIR SIBLING CONTROLS

	Controls	Subjects
No. of cases	50	50
Mean birth order	2.02	2.20
Duration of pregnancy (wks)	40.2	40.4
Mean birth weight ± SD	3.4066	2.8464
	±0.2711	±0.4160

Table 6–2. FACTORS IN INTRAUTERINE IMPOVERISHMENT IN FIFTY CASES

	Percent of cases
Poor diet	10
Weight gain failure	18
Mother small-for-dates	4
Rapid succession of pregnancy	14
Plural pregnancy	4
Acetonuria with or without diabetes	0
Proteinuria	2
Drugs (heroin, amphetamines, phenothiazines)	10

POOR DIET

The impact of malnutrition on brain development has been the subject of much study in recent years and will not be recapitulated here. Data reported by Moghissi *et al.* (17) and Caldwell and Churchill (3) present findings on nutrient effects on mammalian learning.

WEIGHT GAIN FAILURE

Niswander *et al.* (19) have demonstrated that weight gain failure, where the variable is probably a general reflection of undernutrition, affects birth weight. In a prospective study of siblings, Churchill (6) showed an association between maternal weight gain and IQ in sibling pairs.

MOTHER SMALL-FOR-DATE

A few studies in animals have suggested that a mother who was herself stunted *in utero,* or undernourished in early life, may produce small offspring with poor immunologic competence (4, 11). This interesting factor could be studied in greater detail by comparing children born to twin mothers as contrasted to those born to singleton mothers.

RAPID SUCCESSION OF PREGNANCY

Fourteen percent of the mentally impaired children were products of pregnancy begun within 6 months following the birth of a preceding sibling. In a prospective study of the COLR* data, we had compared birth weights and IQs of children conceived within 3 months of a previous pregnancy to matched controls whose mothers had a 2- to 5-year pregnancy-free interval. The results clearly showed the disadvantage of closely spaced pregnancies (13).

PLURAL PREGNANCY

Plural pregnancy is a well-known source of low weight babies, even in those born at term. Less well known are results of studies showing the risk of mental deficits for twins (9). Our original work has been confirmed by Myrianthopolous (18) using different methods of analysis on the same COLR data file.

ACETONURIA WITH OR WITHOUT DIABETES

The present study does not include any mother with diabetes, and data on acetonuria was not obtainable. However, the results of a previous study on offspring of diabetic mothers shows that those mothers whose diabetes was

*Collaborative study of cerebral palsy, mental retardation, and other neurologic and sensory disorders of childhood, National Institute of Neurologic Disease and Stroke.

not well-controlled, as evidenced by acetonuria, account for children with the deficits in developmental measures (8). Well-controlled diabetic mothers have children with no learning deficits; they tend to have the babies of high birth weight.

Acetonuria in pregnancy in the absence of diabetes also results in offspring with deficits in IQ (7). Acetonuria may be an indicator of undernutrition or periods of fasting.

PROTEINURIA

The mother of one of the infants was studied intensively for proteinuria that remained unexplained. In prospectively collected data of the COLR project, we have previously reported on an association of proteinuria of unexplained origin in mothers and the decreased IQs of their children (20).

DRUGS

The effect on the fetus of drugs taken by the mother during pregnancy has been a difficult problem to assess. Lately, investigators have described mental retardation as an element in a syndrome of babies born to alcoholic mothers (14). Amphetamine, noted in the present study, may cause adverse effects by inhibiting the appetite of the mother.

PLACENTAL INSUFFICIENCY

No plausible etiologic factor for the child's low birth weight and learning disability could be found in a number of the present study cases shown on Table 6–2. The lack of indicators suggests that some factors remain unidentified, or that those are cases where stunting was caused by placental insufficiency. Investigators have indicated placental abnormality as a source of small-for-dates infants (12).

CONCLUSION

There is now general agreement that small-for-dates infants differ from premature ones. Studies show that children with learning disabilities and mental retardation are often small-for-dates infants. The clear association of learning disability and small-for-dates infants points to disturbances occurring during intrauterine life as the source for much, and perhaps the major amount, of depressed mental capacity. The factors studied and presented here and shown to be associated with small full-term infants with deficits in learning functions can all be viewed as having the common effect of diminishing supplies of nutrients to the fetus.

The infant suffering from intrauterine impoverishment is not merely small and so of small concern: it is stunted and has a permanent warp imposed within the fabric of its brain which may be expected to impede learning processes throughout its life. Thus mental retardation, which affects 3% of the population, should be a matter of great concern to obstetricians.

REFERENCES

1. Alm F: The long term prognosis for prematurely born children. A follow-up study of 999 premature boys born in wedlock and of 1002 controls. Acta Paediatr Scand 94:1, 1953

2. Bandera E, Churchill J: Prematurity and neurologic disorders. Henry Ford Hosp Bull 9:414, 1961

3. Caldwell D, Churchill J: Learning ability in the progeny of rats administered a protein deficient diet during the second half of gestation. Neurology (Minneap) 17:95, 1967

4. Chandra R: Antibody formation in first and second generation offspring of nutritionally deprived rats. Science 190:289, 1975

5. Churchill J: Spastic diplegia of premature birth. Henry Ford Hosp Bull 4:257, 1959

6. Churchill J: Maternal weight gain and IQ of siblings. Lansing, MI, Proc Mich Med Soc, 1966

7. Churchill J, Berendes H: Intelligence of children whose mothers had acetonuria during pregnancy. In Perinatal Factors Affecting Human Development. Washington DC, Pan American Health Organization, WHO, 1969, pp 30–35

8. Churchill J, Berendes H, Nemore J: Neuropsychological deficits in children of diabetic mothers. Am J Obstet Gynecol 105:257, 1969

9. Churchill J, Henderson W: Perinatal factors affecting fetal development—twin pregnancy. In Moghissi KS (ed): Birth Defects and Fetal Development. Springfield, Ill, CC Thomas, 1974, pp 69–76

10. Churchill J, Neff M, Caldwell D: Birthweight and intelligence. Obstet Gynecol 28:425, 1966

11. Cowley J, Griesel R: The development of second generation low protein rats. J Genet Psychol 103:233, 1963

12. Gruenwald P: Chronic fetal distress and placental insufficiency. Biol Neonate 5:215, 1963

13. Holley W, Rosenbaum A, Churchill J: Effect of rapid succession of pregnancy. In Perinatal Factors Affecting Human Development. Washington DC, Pan American Health Organization, WHO, 1969, pp 41–44

14. Jones K, Smith DW, Streissguth AP, Myrianthopoulos NC: Outcome in offspring of chronic alcoholic women. Lancet 1:1076, 1974

15. Little W: On the influence of abnormal parturition, difficult labor, premature birth, and asphyxia neonatorum on the mental and physical condition of the child, especially in relation to deformities. Lancet 2:378, 1861

16. Macdonald A: Intelligence in children of very low birth weight. Br J Prev Soc Med 18:59, 1964

17. Moghissi KS, Churchill J, Kurrie D: Relationship of maternal amino acids and proteins to fetal growth and mental development. Am J Obstet Gynecol 123:398, 1975

18. Myrianthopolous NC: A survey of twins in the population of a prospective collaborative study. Acta Genet Med Gemellol (Roma) 19:15, 1970

19. Niswander KS, Singer J, Westphal M, Weiss W: Weight gain during pregnancy and prepregnancy weight. Association with birth weight of term gestation. Obstet Gynecol 33:482, 1969

20. Rosenbaum A, Churchill J, Shakhashiri Z, Moody R: Neuropsychologic outcome of children whose mothers had proteinuria during pregnancy. Obstet Gynecol 33:118, 1969
21. Willerman L, Churchill J: Intelligence and birthweight in identical twins. Child Dev 12:623, 1967

Chapter 7

Amino Acid Sources for the Fetus

Roy M. Pitkin

A fundamental requisite for the extraordinarily complex process of growth and development of the mammalian fetus is the provision of various metabolic substrates. The α-amino nitrogen compounds—proteins, peptides, and amino acids—are particularly important, for they represent the essential building blocks in the laying down of new tissues, the hallmark of growth.

α-Amino nitrogen compounds, as all other nutrients utilized by the fetus, are provided ultimately by the mother. They reach the fetus by two routes, the principal of which is via the placenta. Amino acids represent the major form in which placental transfer occurs, although transport of peptides and (to a lesser extent) macromolecular protein occurs as well. Amniotic fluid contains amino acids and protein, and its ingestion by the fetus represents a secondary source of α-amino nitrogen which, while quantitatively smaller than the transplacental source, nevertheless appears to play an important role in fetal growth and development.

PLACENTAL TRANSFER

CHARACTERISTICS

Placental transport of amino acids has long been a popular area for investigation. Numerous studies utilizing *in vivo* and *in vitro* methodology in a variety of species have been done. From the large number of such reported studies, certain characteristics of amino acid transfer by the placenta emerge (15). Chief among these is the observation that net maternal–fetal transfer occurs for the most part against a concentration gradient, *i.e.*, from a lower level in maternal blood to a higher level in fetal blood. The rather remarkable degree of stereospecificity, by which the naturally occurring L forms are transported substantially more rapidly than D forms, represents another characteristic.

Still another is the lack of binding proteins in fetal plasma to account for fetal accumulation. Moreover, transfer of one amino acid can be inhibited by increased concentration of similar amino acids, presumably by competition for specific common transfer sites. Finally, increasing maternal levels above a certain

75

point causes no further elevation in fetal levels, suggesting saturation of a transport system.

On the basis of these considerations—transfer against a gradient, stereospecificity, lack of fetal binding proteins, competitive inhibition, and a saturation effect—placental transfer of amino acids is generally regarded as occurring by an active transport system.

MATERNAL AND FETAL LEVELS

In general, maternal plasma levels of amino acids decline during pregnancy. However, there is considerable variation in the patterns of individual amino acids (Table 7–1). For some the fall occurs progressively throughout gestation; for others it is limited to early or (in a few cases) late pregnancy. In the case of at least three amino acids (asparagine, glutamic acid, and histidine), concentrations change little if any. The mechanism or mechanisms responsible for the generally declining plasma amino acid levels in pregnancy is unknown. Urinary excretion of amino acids is substantially increased during pregnancy (4), but the pattern and timing do not exhibit close correlation with changing plasma levels. Similarly, the pattern does not resemble that anticipated with hemodilution. Placental transfer is unlikely as a cause since much of the decline occurs in early pregnancy, when fetal demands are small. Hormonal factors may play a role since some degree of variation occurs during the menstrual cycle and changes similar to those during pregnancy are encountered with estrogen and progesterone treatment. Whatever the mechanism, the response seems to be a physiologic one (17).

That plasma levels of amino acids in the fetus generally exceed those in the pregnant woman has been appreciated for nearly 60 years (7). As noted previously, this relationship represents part of the evidence suggesting an active placental transport system. The fetal–maternal ratio of individual amino acids generally ranges from 1.5 to 3, with a slight tendency toward lowering of the ratio as pregnancy progresses (3). Teleologically, such a transplacental gradient favoring the fetus has certain obvious advantages in insuring provision of adequate substrate levels for growth and development. However, that such a set of circumstances is not invariably favorable is illustrated by the now-classic studies

Table 7–1. MATERNAL PLASMA AMINO ACID LEVELS DURING PREGNANCY*

Progressive decline through pregnancy	Decline first half, constant last half	Constant first half, decline last half	Essentially no change
Alanine	Cystine	Arginine	Asparagine
Glycine	Lysine	Isolencine	Glutamic acid
Serine	Methionine	Phenylalanine	Histidine
Taurine	Ornithine		
Valine	Proline		
	Threonine		
	Tyrosine		

*Hytten FE, Cheyne GA: J Obstet Gynaecol Br Commonw. 79:424, 1972

of Kerr *et al.* (5) and Kerr and Waisman (6), who found that the transplacental gradient for phenylalanine was maintained in monkeys fed a diet high in that amino acid during pregnancy. The infants born to these monkeys had high phenylalanine levels and were slow to learn simple tasks, symptoms apparently corresponding to those of the well-known clinical syndrome of maternal phenylketonuria.

The question of whether the transplacental gradient for amino acids is maintained in the face of maternal hyperaminoacidemia, in addition to its importance in understanding placental physiology, has assumed clinical significance with the relatively recent advent of total parenteral nutrition. We have examined this matter in pregnant rhesus monkeys, a species with a hemochorial placenta virtually identical in both structure and function to that of humans. Catheterization of the interplacental vessels permitted sequential sampling of fetal blood with the fetus *in utero* and the amniotic sac intact. For these studies, pregnant animals were infused with a total parenteral nutrition solution of 5% mixed synthetic amino acids. The solution—which contained a total of 16 amino acids, including the 8 regarded as essential—was infused at a constant rate of infusion over 8 to 10 hours. Simultaneous maternal and fetal plasma samples taken at hourly intervals were analyzed for amino acid composition. Figure 7–1 illustrates the fetal–maternal gradients for selected amino acids before and after 6 hours of infusion. The gradient for three amino acids (cystine, leucine, and lysine) increased, indicating that fetal levels were raised to a proportionately greater degree than maternal levels. In the case of three others (isoleucine, phenylalanine, and arginine), the gradient fell only slightly and probably not to a statistically significant degree. The gradient for all other amino acids (illustrated in Figure 7–1 by glycine, proline, and histidine) declined with elevation of the maternal levels, indicating somewhat of a "blunting" effect on the fetal side of the placenta. Thus, while induced maternal hyperaminoacidemia was generally reflected in elevated fetal levels, the most frequent pattern observed was that of a somewhat disproportionately smaller increase in the fetal, compared with maternal, response.

SELECTIVE TRANSFER

Even among the natural L forms, the placenta exhibits a considerable degree of selectivity with respect to transfer of individual amino acids. Probably each compound has a different rate of transfer, and for some the placenta is virtually impermeable. In *in vitro* studies, Schneider and Dancis (12) examined uptake, accumulation, and release of ten amino acids in human placental slices. The acidic amino acids—glutamic and aspartic acids, and to a lesser extent serine—exhibited rapid uptake, extensive intracellular accumulation, and negligible efflux. By contrast, neutral and basic amino acids were taken up more slowly and accumulated intracellularly to a much lesser degree because of a rapid efflux. The rate of efflux for leucine was especially rapid, since the ratio of intracellular to extracellular concentration of this compound remained below one. From these observations, it would be anticipated that leucine would be transferred very

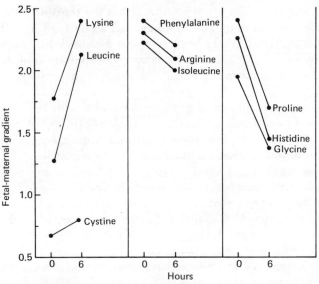

Fig. 7–1. Fetal–maternal gradients at 0 and 6 hours of maternal infusion of amino acid mixture.

rapidly; other neutral and basic amino acids rapidly; and glutamate, aspartate, and serine to a minimal degree.

In vivo confirmation of these observations is available with respect to glutamate and aspartate. We recently reported studies of placental transfer of glutamate and its metabolites in pregnant rhesus monkeys infused with varying doses of the amino acid (13). Maternal blood, fetal blood, and amniotic fluid were sampled sequentially. As indicated in Figure 7–2, maternal infusions of approximately 0.2 g/kg maternal weight produced maternal plasma glutamate levels of 50–100 μmol/dl (10 to 20 times normal values), but fetal plasma levels did not change. With maternal infusion at 0.4 g/kg, maternal levels reached 280 μ mol/dl (70 times normal) and some degree of placental transfer apparently occurred, producing fetal values as high as 44 μmol/dl (10 times normal). These observations suggest that the hemochorial placenta is essentially impermeable to glutamate at anything less than massively elevated maternal levels. They further suggest something resembling a threshold phenomenon for maternal–fetal transfer at a maternal level around 250 μmol/dl, perhaps by high levels of glutamate that in some way temporarily disrupt the placental membranes.

Insight into the metabolism of glutamate in pregnancy was gained by infusions containing tracer amounts of added 3,4-^{14}C-glutamate. Figure 7–3 illustrates the radioactivity profile of glutamate metabolites during and following maternal infusion in a representative experiment. During the infusion, glutamate accounted for most of the radioactivity in the maternal plasma. Some radioactivity during the infusion, and most of it after the infusion, was present in two ninhydrin-negative compounds identified as glucose and lactate. Smaller

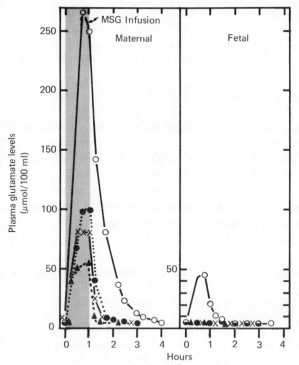

Figure 7–2. Maternal and fetal plasma glutamate levels with maternal glutamate infusion at several dosage levels: 0.15 g/kg, *solid triangles;* 0.17–0.19 g/kg, *x;* 0.22 g/kg, *solid circles;* 0.4 g/kg, *open circles.* (Stegink LD, Pitkin RM, Reynolds WA, et al.: Am J Obstet Gynecol 122:70, 1975)

Fig. 7–3. Radioactivity profile of glutamate metabolites with maternal glutamate infusion 0.22 g/kg. (Stegink LD, Pitkin RM, Reynolds WA, et al.: Am J Obstet Gynecol 122:70, 1975)

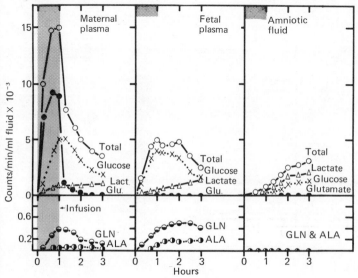

quantities of radioactivity occurred in association with two glutamate-derived amino acids—glutamine and alanine. By contrast, most of the radioactivity in the fetus represented glucose and lactate, with essentially none in glutamate. Radioactive lactate and glucose were also transferred to the amniotic fluid.

From these studies involving simultaneously determined chemical and radioactive levels with glutamate infusion, a clear picture of glutamate metabolism in the pregnant primate emerges. Transfer to the fetus does not occur at maternal levels less than extreme. Instead, glutamate is metabolized to glucose and lactate in the mother, and these metabolites, as well as small amounts of glutamate-derived amino acids, cross the placenta quite readily. But glutamate itself is not transferred under anything remotely resembling normal circumstances.

Virtually the same situation applied with aspartate, the other dicarboxylic amino acid in plasma. As illustrated in Figure 7–4, maternal aspartate infusions of 0.1 g/kg produced maximal maternal levels of approximately 60 μmol/dl (100 times normal) but no change in fetal levels. Under conditions of extreme elevation of maternal plasma levels (575 μmol/dl or 1000 times normal), some degree of transfer to the fetus occurred.

In summary: The placenta is capable of transmitting the majority of amino

Figure 7–4. Maternal and fetal plasma aspartate levels with maternal aspartate infusion with 0.4g/kg *(open circles)* and 0.1 g/kg *(solid circles)* aspartate.

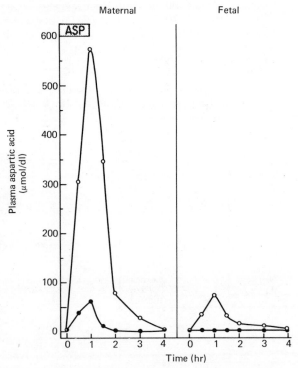

acids with facility, apparently by an active transport process. Glutamic and aspartic acids represent important exceptions, and cystine and cysteine may also be exceptions (14).

AMNIOTIC FLUID INGESTION

AMINO ACID AND PROTEIN LEVELS

Both amino acids and proteins are present in amniotic fluid and represent potential sources of α-amino nitrogen available to the fetus. Whether the amino acids in amniotic fluid are derived from maternal plasma or fetal urine is a matter of some controversy. In any event, the levels in general decline quite remarkably during late pregnancy. With the exception of cystine, ethanolamine, glutamine, and taurine, by term the concentrations fall to half or less of those of the first half of gestation (8).

On the basis of electrophoretic patterns, it appears that most of the protein in amniotic fluid originates directly from the maternal plasma (1). Total protein levels in amniotic fluid decline during late pregnancy, though in a somewhat different pattern and perhaps to a lesser extent than amino acid levels. During the second trimester, there appears to be a slight rise which is followed by a progressive downward trend from 24 weeks to and beyond term. For example, mean values of 0.64 g/dl at 20–24 weeks and 0.28 g/dl at 37–40 weeks have been reported (11). Albumin accounts for most of the decline with other protein fractions changing inconsistently (16).

FETAL INGESTION AND METABOLISM

The fetus normally swallows amniotic fluid in amounts averaging 500 ml/day near term (10). This phenomenon coupled with declining amniotic fluid protein levels suggests a possible nutritive function for amniotic fluid during late intrauterine life. Such an hypothesis is further suggested by observations that infants with congenital malformations interfering with swallowing are particularly likely to exhibit intrauterine growth retardation (2).

Ingestion and metabolism of amniotic fluid protein by the fetus has recently been studied in rhesus monkeys in which a biologically synthesized ^{35}S-labeled protein was injected into the amniotic sac at timed intervals prior to delivery (9). Approximately half of the amniotic fluid protein content was cleared per day by fetal swallowing. Proteolysis along the fetal alimentary tract and the fate of labeled amino acids thus liberated was examined.

Figure 7–5 illustrates the radioactivity in the fetal gut contents following injection of labeled protein into the amniotic sac. Progressive proteolysis along the course of the small intestine is evident, with amino acid radioactivity highest in the ileum on days 1–2 after injection. By days 5–7 after injection, the amino acid radioactivity was highest in the stomach, reflecting continued fetal swallowing of amniotic fluid which by that time had accumulated substantial quantities of amino acids from fetal excretion. Radioactive protein levels in the alimentary tract contents exhibited a course exactly opposite that of amino acid levels. Early, they were highest in the stomach, reflecting ingestion of labeled protein, while later they were highest in the distal small intestine, apparently as a result of desquamation of cells containing protein synthesized in the gut wall.

Amino acids liberated by proteolysis in the fetal alimentary tract were absorbed into fetal plasma where, as illustrated in Figure 7–6, they equilibrated with amniotic fluid and maternal plasma. These amino acids were then utilized in protein synthesis in a variety of fetal tissues.

Figure 7–7 summarizes the metabolism of ingested amniotic fluid protein. Swallowed protein is hydrolyzed in the fetal alimentary tract and absorbed as individual amino acids or small peptides. These may be 1) utilized in protein synthesis in the gut wall, part of which is later reexcreted into the lumen; 2) transported by blood to be incorporated into protein in any fetal tissue; 3) transferred across the placenta to the mother; or 4) excreted into the amniotic fluid to be swallowed again and recycled.

Thus, ingested amniotic fluid protein may play several physiologic roles in

Fig. 7–5. Radioactivity in fetal alimentary tract contents after injection of ³⁵S-protein into amniotic sac. Top (amino acids) refers to trichloracetic acid (TCA)-soluble radioactivity. Bottom (protein) refers to TCA-insoluble radioactivity. stomach, *S;* duodenum, *D;* jejunum, *J;* ileum, *I;* colon, *C.* (Pitkin RM, Reynolds WA: Am J Obstet Gynecol 423:356, 1975)

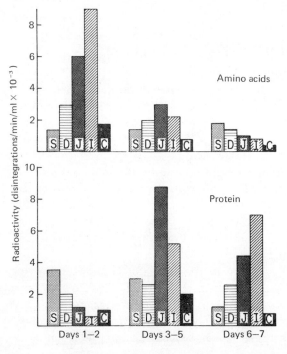

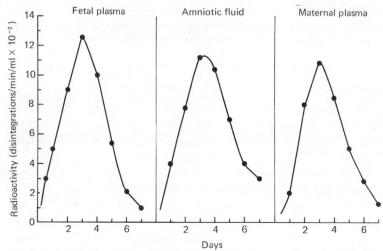

Fig. 7–6. Radioactivity in amino acids in fetal plasma, amniotic fluid, and maternal plasma after injection of ^{35}S-protein into amniotic sac. (Pitkin RM, Reynolds WA: Am J Obstet Gynecol 123:356, 1975)

Fig. 7–7. Fetal metabolism of amniotic fluid protein.

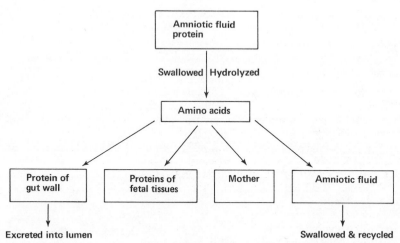

fetal growth; however, any such role is admittedly small in comparison to the transplacental source of nitrogen. Using known values for the amniotic fluid protein concentration and volume of fetal swallowing, it can be calculated that this mechanism could provide some 10%–15% of estimated nitrogen requirements in the term human fetus. Though this may not seem significant quantitatively, it may represent an important role physiologically in enzyme induction or other mechanisms necessary in preparing the gastrointestinal tract for its nutritional function after birth. Finally, the demonstration that amniotic fluid protein is metabolized and utilized by the fetus suggests the possibility of therapeutic use of intraamniotic injection of nutrients in abnormal states such as fetal growth retardation.

SUMMARY

The α-amino nitrogen essential for fetal growth and development is provided by two mechanisms. The principal source is transplacental and involves active transport of amino acids from mother to fetus against a concentration gradient. With induction of maternal hyperaminoacidemia, the gradient for most amino acids tends to be lessened slightly, resulting in a somewhat lesser degree of fetal than maternal plasma response. Thus, amino acids in general are transported with facility, insuring adequacy from the fetal point of view. The rates of transfer for individual amino acids are probably specific for each compound. Moreover, the dicarboxylic amino acids (glutamic and aspartic acids) are not transported by the hemochorial placenta, and their presence in the fetus is due entirely to fetal synthesis from other amino acids or precursors.

A secondary source of fetal amino acids is ingested amniotic fluid. Amniotic fluid contains both amino acids and protein, and the fetal alimentary tract is capable of proteolysis. Amino acids from either amniotic fluid or hydrolyzed amniotic fluid protein are absorbed from the fetal gut and are available for fetal protein synthesis.

REFERENCES

1. Abbas TM, Tovey JE: Proteins of the liquor amnii. Br Med J 1:476, 1960
2. David TJ, O'Callaghan SE: Oerophageal atresia in the southwest of England. J Med Genet 12:1, 1975
3. Ghadimi H, Pecora P: Free amino acids of cord plasma as compared with maternal plasma during pregnancy. Pediatrics 30: 500, 1964
4. Hytten FE, Cheyne GA: The aminoaciduria of pregnancy. J Obstet Gynaecol., Br Commonw 79: 424, 1972
5. Kerr GR, Chamove AS, Harlow HF, Waisman HA: Fetal PKU: The effect of maternal hyperphenylalaninemia during pregnancy in the rhesus monkey (Macaca mulatta). Pediatrics 42: 27, 1968
6. Kerr JR, Waisman HA: Transplacental ratios of serum free amino acids during pregnancy in the rhesus monkey. In Nyhan WL (ed): Amino Acid Metabolism and Genetic Variation. New York, McGraw–Hill, 1967, p 429
7. Morse A: The amino acid nitrogen of the blood in cases of normal and complicated pregnancy and also in the newborn infant. Johns Hopkins Med J 28: 199, 1917
8. O'Neill RT, Morrow G III, Hammel D, Auerbach VH, Barness LA: Diagnostic significance of amniotic fluid amino acids. Obstet Gynecol 37:550, 1971
9. Pitkin RM, Reynolds WA: Fetal ingestion and metabolism of amniotic fluid protein. Am J Obstet Gynecol 123: 356, 1975
10. Pritchard JA: Deglutition by normal and anencephalic fetuses. Obstet Gynecol 25: 289, 1965
11. Queenan JT, Gadow EC, Bachner P, Kubarych SF: Amniotic fluid proteins in normal and Rh-sensitized pregnancies. Am J Obstet Gynecol 108: 406, 1970

12. Schneider H, Dancis J: Amino acid transport in human placental slices. Am J Obstet Gynecol 120: 1092, 1974
13. Stegink LD, Pitkin RM, Reynolds WA, Filer LJ Jr, Boaz DP, Brummel MC: Placental transfer of glutamate and its metabolites in the primate. Am J Obstet Gynecol 122: 70, 1975
14. Sturman JA, Niemann WH, Gaull EB: Metabolism of ^{35}S-methionine and ^{35}S-cystine in the pregnant rhesus monkey. Biol Neonate 22:16, 1973
15. Szabo AJ, Grimaldi RD: The metabolism of the placenta. Levine R, Luff R (eds): In Advances in Metabolic Disorders, Vol 4. New York, Academic Press, 1970, p 217
16. Touchstone JC, Glazer LG, Bolognese RJ, Corson SL: Gestational age and amniotic fluid protein patterns. Am J Obstet Gynecol 114: 58, 1972
17. Young M: Placental transport of free amino acids. In Jonxis JHP, Visser HKA, Troelstra JA (eds): Metabolic Processes in the Foetus and Newborn Infant. Leiden, HE Stenfert Kroese NV, 1971, p 97

Chapter 8

Relationship of Maternal Amino Acids and Proteins to Infant Growth and Mental Development

Kamran S. Moghissi

Numerous animal experiments suggest that inadequate or deficient maternal nutrition during pregnancy leads to intrauterine stunting and impairment of fetal brain development. Protein and other nutritional deficiencies in rodents lead to retardation of growth, increased mortality, lowered intelligence, and physical and behavioral abnormalities (2, 3, 6, 7, 28, 33). Caloric restriction of rats from day 10 to 20 of pregnancy results in a significant decrease in body weight, placental weight, cerebral weight, and cerebral DNA and cerebral protein levels of offspring at birth (44). Animals born of protein-restricted mothers demonstrate a permanent impairment in their ability to utilize nitrogen and remain with a deficit in total brain cell number at weaning (42) even if they are nursed by normal foster mothers receiving adequate nutrition.

Other related studies have clearly demonstrated that the physical growth of the brain can be seriously restricted by comparatively mild undernutrition during the periods of its fastest growth and that such restrictions have certain permanent sequelae. The greatest increase in mass in the human fetus, particularly that of its brain, occurs during the last few weeks of gestation and continues during the first few months after birth.

Unlike investigations in animals, studies in women are fraught with considerable difficulties since the experimental conditions cannot be precisely regulated. Human malnutrition is commonly associated with such factors as poverty, lack of education, social deprivation, and increased incidence of infection and chronic diseases. It is difficult to dissociate the mutual influence that these factors exert upon each other. Despite these handicaps, much indirect data have been gathered indicating that the physical and mental well-being of infants subjected to malnutrition during pregnancy may be affected in a manner similar to those observed in other mammalian species.

Conditions which are known to make greater demands on maternal nutritional reserve such as twinning (19) and rapid succession of pregnancies (20) are associated with low-birth-weight infants who have lower IQs (Table 8–1).

Substantial evidence linking directly maternal malnutrition to intrauterine growth retardation and subsequent mental or behavioral deficiency in the infants is still lacking. Furthermore, there are no reliable parameters by which to

Table 8–1. CONDITIONS WHICH HAVE DELETERIOUS EFFECTS
ON FETAL GROWTH *IN UTERO* (BIRTH WEIGHT)

Twining
Maternal acetonuria during pregnancy
  (third trimester)
Rapid succession of pregnancies
Number of previous pregnancies
Birth weight last pregnancy
Prepregnancy weight
Smoking

identify potentially malnourished fetuses from true prematures or those with growth retardation resulting from other causes.

In this chapter, the protein and amino acid changes during pregnancy in the maternal and fetal blood and the amniotic fluid are briefly reviewed, and the effect of protein deprivation during human gestation is discussed by comparing changes of maternal blood levels of individual amino acids, blood proteins, and certain maternal factors with infant growth at birth and mental development at 8 months of age. Most of the data resulted from prospective studies performed during the last few years at Wayne State University.

PROTEINS AND AMINO ACID CHANGES DURING PREGNANCY

SERUM PROTEINS

During pregnancy there is a positive nitrogen balance to meet the requirements of the fetus and the growth of the reproductive tract. There may also be a retention of nitrogen for other maternal organs such as the alimentary tract and liver. The amount of retained nitrogen has been estimated to be between 1.-17–1.3 g/day (22, 46) and exceeds fetal needs by a considerable margin if protein intake is adequate.

Pregnancy brings about considerable changes in serum protein levels. There is a progressive decline in total protein and albumin concentrations and a steady decrease in the albumin/globulin ratio. Late in puerperium, total protein and albumin levels return to prepregnancy levels, and the albumin/globulin ratio assumes the prepregnancy relationship. Serum concentrations of many globulins are also altered in the course of gestation (Table 8–2). A pregnancy zone protein which migrates electrophoretically in α_2-globulin region has been observed in the sera of the majority of pregnant women (1, 4, 26, 38, 39).

Large molecular weight proteins are selectively transported across the placental barrier in varying amounts. Transplacental transmission of proteins was investigated by Gitlin *et al.* (12, 16, 17), who labeled proteins with ^{125}I or ^{131}I, administered them to pregnant women by a single intravenous injection and studied their distribution in maternal and fetal blood and amniotic fluid.

The disappearance of labeled albumin from the plasma of pregnant women was similar to that observed in nonpregnant women.

Labeled proteins disappeared rather rapidly from the maternal circulation.

Table 8–2. ALTERATION OF MATERNAL SERUM PROTEIN LEVELS DURING PREGNANCY

Proteins	Changes during pregnancy
Total proteins	Decreased (26)
Albumin	Decreased (26)
Albumin/globulin ratio	Decreased (26)
α_1-Globulins	Increased (26)
α_1-Lipoprotein	Unchanged (4)
α_1-Antitrypsin	Increased (4)
α_1-Glycoprotein (easily precipitable)	Increased (4)
Gc globulin	Increased (4)
α_2-globulins	Increased (26)
Haptoglobulin	Unchanged (4)
Ceruloplasmin	Increased (4)
α_2-Macroglobulin	Unchanged (4)
β-Globulins	Increased (26)
Transferrin	Increased (4)
Thermopexin	Unchanged (4)
Fibrinogen	Increased (26)
β_1-Lipoprotein	Unchanged (4)
β_1-AC (C'3)	Unchanged (4)
γ-Globulin	Decreased (26)
Specific proteins	
α_1-Fetoprotein	Marked increase (39)
Pregnancy zone protein (α_2)	Appearance & marked increase (38)

Reference numbers are given in parentheses.

This was primarily due to the rapid diffusion of the proteins from the vascular system into the maternal interstitial space and not due to maternal–fetal transfer. The plasma concentration of labeled albumin in the fetus relative to that in the mother increased with time during the study period of approximately 33 days. The rate of increase in the fetal plasma concentrations of α_1-acid glycoprotein, albumin, transferrin, and fibrinogen was inversely proportional to the square root of their molecular weight. Thus, the evidence strongly suggested that these proteins passed through the maternal–fetal barrier into the fetal circulation by diffusion.

Individual placentas may vary widely in their relative permeability to a given plasma protein. In some women, relatively little labeled albumin passes into the fetal plasma as compared to the maternal–fetal transfer of the same protein in other women.

The maternal transfer of IgG is much more efficient than that of the other plasma proteins such as α_1-acid glycoprotein, albumin, and transferrin which have smaller molecules than those of IgG. Human IgG is believed to cross placental barrier by two mechanisms, i.e., diffusion and the carrier, (receptor-mediated), process which is inhibited by its own substrate, human IgG. At high maternal levels of IgG the diffusion process is predominantly operative; whereas, at low maternal levels the receptor or carrier process is more efficient. This dual mechanism maintains a relatively stable level of IgG in the fetus even though there may be a considerable variation in maternal concentration of this protein.

Fetal Protein Synthesis

At 29 days of gestation the liver of the human embryo is capable of synthesizing many plasma proteins including prealbumin, albumin, α-fetoprotein, α_1-antitrypsin, α_1-acid glycoprotein, α_2-macroglobulin, C'1 esterase inhibitor, β_{1c}-lipoprotein, hemopexin, and transferrin (13). At 4½–5 weeks of gestation, the hepatic lobes of the embryo are recognizable, and the liver can also synthesize ceruloplasmin. By 5½ weeks of gestation, hepatic synthesis of fibrinogen is initiated. IgM synthesis begins about 10½ weeks, and that of IgG between 11–12 weeks of gestation (14). Between 38 days and 16 weeks of gestation, the serum concentration of IgG in the human conceptus is approximately 5%–8% of that in the mother. Only minute amounts of IgG are produced by the fetus before 16 weeks of gestation, and virtually all of the IgG found in the fetal serum prior to 16 weeks of pregnancy is diffused from the maternal circulation. After 17 weeks, significant synthesis of IgG can occur in the fetal spleen, giving rise to slight elevation of fetal serum IgG. After 22 weeks of gestation there is an abrupt rise in fetal serum IgG concentration that reaches levels approximately equal to those of the mother. Since during this period the fetus synthesizes IgG at a rate of less than 1% of that in the adult per unit of weight, this rapid increase in fetal IgG concentration must be due to a sudden increase in placental permeability to IgG. The increase in permeability of placental barrier appears to be selective for IgG and not due to a general increase in permeability resulting from the loss of a cell layer in the placenta (12).

IgM, unlike IgG, does not cross the placenta, and although the fetus can synthesize IgM (13), the amount normally produced during intrauterine life is quite small. At birth the level of IgM is very low and is related to birth weight and gestational age, being higher in larger and more mature infants (40).

AMINO ACIDS

It is generally accepted that the free α-amino acid concentration is reduced in the maternal plasma during pregnancy (43). The total free amino acid nitrogen is about 25% lower than in the plasma of nonpregnant women. The reduction in concentration is not the same for all amino acids (45) (see Ch. 7, Amino Acid Sources for the Fetus). The decrease in maternal plasma free amino acid is already present early in the second trimester, and the levels remain constant during the subsequent course of gestation and during the early postpartum period. Reid et al. (35) found that, at 7–18 weeks of gestation, the levels of ten plasma amino acids were significantly lower than corresponding nonpregnancy levels. Six other amino acids showed a tendency to be lower, whereas taurine, aspartic acid, glutamic acid, leucine and phenylalanine showed no significant change. Between 36 and 40 weeks of gestation the plasma amino acid levels were either decreased or did not change from those of the nonpregnant control group. The only exceptions were glutamic acid levels, which showed a significant increase, and taurine and leucine levels, which showed a trend to decrease from early to late pregnancy.

Amino acids pass freely and rapidly across the placenta by active transport and have a higher concentration in fetal than in maternal plasma (10, 11, 25).

It has been shown that the ratio of essential amino acid concentrations in the umbilical vein to those in the maternal anticubital vein is lower in pregnancies complicated by intrauterine growth retardation compared to the normal (37). Increased aminoaciduria during pregnancy is well-documented (29).

AMNIOTIC FLUID

Proteins

A progressive decrease in the amount of proteins in amniotic fluid is observed in the course of gestation. During the first 6 months of pregnancy the levels vary between 0.6 and 1.8 mg/100 ml. A plateau is reached prior to 32 weeks, after which there is a progressive decrease (Figs. 8–1 and 8–2). Higher levels of proteins have been found when the fetus has been critically affected by erythroblastosis. An inverse relationship between amniotic fluid protein levels and infant birth weight has been demonstrated (27). Electrophoretic studies of the amniotic fluid proteins have shown the presence of 21 protein bands among which prealbumin, albumin, α_1-globulins, α_2-globulins (including ceruloplasmin and transferrin) and immunoglobulins (IgA and IgG) have been identified in all samples of amniotic fluid near term. Alpha$_2$-haptoglobulin and α_2-macroglobulin were also observed in some specimens. At term, amniotic fluid contains approximately 20.5 mg/100 ml of protein of which albumin forms 60%; ceruloplasmin, 1.5%; transferrin, 11.6%; IgA, 0.1%; and IgG, 11.0% (8).

Source of Amniotic Fluid Proteins

The source of amniotic fluid proteins has been a subject of controversy for many years. To explore the origin and fate of amniotic fluid proteins, Gitlin *et al.* (12, 15) injected labeled albumin (molecular weight 68,000), IgG and IgA (molecular weight 165,000), chorionic gonadotropin (molecular weight 20,000), and growth hormone (molecular weight 29,000) intraamniotically to pregnant women at 34–40 weeks of gestation and during labor.

The half-life of iodoproteins was prolonged when pregnancy was complicated by intrauterine fetal death. Gitlin *et al.* found that the concentration of endogenous albumin, IgG, IgA, and transferrin in amniotic fluid during the study period did not vary more than 25% from their initial levels and that the amniotic fluid protein turnover seemed to be in a relatively steady state in that a given protein being cleared from amniotic fluid was replaced by an equivalent amount of the same protein entering the amniotic fluid. In nonlaboring pregnant women, approximately 63% of amniotic fluid protein was turned over per day; during labor, it averaged 90%/day. In women with dead fetuses, protein turnover was only 12%. The volume of amniotic fluid cleared of protein daily in those women not in labor ranged from 200–575 ml. Labeled proteins were found in gastric aspirates of the living infants at delivery, indicating fetal swallowing of proteins.

These studies suggest that amniotic fluid proteins originate from both mother

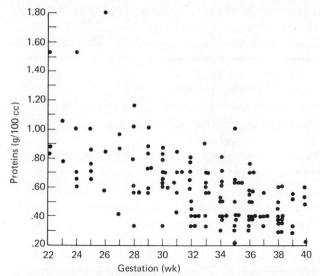

Fig. 8–1. Amniotic fluid protein content showing a progressive decrease. (Mandelbaum B, Evans TN: Am J Obstet Gynecol 104:365, 1969)

Fig. 8–2. Serial determinations of amniotic fluid proteins. (Mandelbaum B, Evans TN: Am J Obstet Gynecol 104:365, 1969)

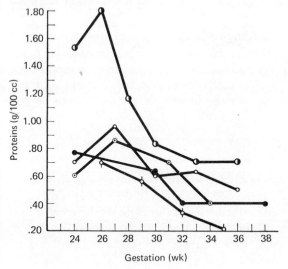

and fetus. The bulk of the amniotic fluid proteins come directly or indirectly from the mother, but fetal urinary proteins also contribute to the pool. A significant fraction of amniotic fluid IgG comes from fetal urine. Even this originates indirectly from maternal serum via placental transfer and fetal serum. Alpha$_1$-fetoprotein present in the amniotic fluid, however, is almost exclusively of fetal origin and is passed into the amniotic fluid via fetal urine or possibly other routes (21). The major process involved in amniotic fluid protein clearance is fetal swallowing. The absorption of intact proteins from amniotic fluid by fetal lung, cord, or skin appears to be negligible.

All of the proteins leaving amniotic fluid are not cleared by fetal swallowing; approximately 10%–15% are probably cleared by diffusion through fetal membranes.

Fetal Swallowing and Its Importance

It is well known that as early as 12 weeks of gestation the fetus is capable of swallowing and concentrating labeled proteins in its gastrointestinal tract. Lev and Orlic (23) injected horseradish peroxidase (a macromolecular protein with molecular weight of about 40,000) into the amniotic cavity of pregnant monkeys and showed that the monkey fetal intestine has the capacity to take up macromolecular protein contained within swallowed amniotic fluid. Studies of amniotic fluid orosomucoid and Gc globulin by the sensitive method of phenotyping have shown that adult-type plasma proteins found in amniotic fluid are almost entirely of maternal origin (21).

The amniotic fluid protein swallowed by the fetus is subsequently hydrolyzed to amino acids, absorbed and utilized by the fetus for the synthesis of body proteins. Only a fraction of the ingested and absorbed proteins is subsequently excreted into the amniotic fluid. Thus, amniotic fluid proteins swallowed by the fetus are not merely recycled but are, for the most part, a contribution by the mother to fetal metabolism.

Amino Acids

In the amniotic fluid between 7–18 weeks of gestation, the concentration of most of the amino acids are significantly increased compared to the concentrations in the maternal plasma, but the concentrations are not significantly different when compared to those in nonpregnancy plasma. At term (36–40 weeks), Reid et al. (35) found that 15 amino acids were lower in amniotic fluid as compared to maternal plasma and six others showed no difference. Levy and Montag (24), showed also that free amino acids in human full-term amniotic fluid were identical to those present in maternal and umbilical cord serum, but the concentration of the 23 free amino acids detected in amniotic fluid were 50–75% of the respective concentrations in maternal serum. Dallaire et al. (5) found that the concentration of eight amino acids decreased toward the end of pregnancy in amniotic fluid; thirteen amino acids showed no significant change from the 10th to the 40th week of gestation, while ten were present in trace amounts during the same period. Alanine was measurable both in early and late pregnancy. The mean serine glycine and arginine concentrations showed no significant variation from the tenth week to term. Amino acid concentrations in amniotic fluid of twin gestations is markedly increased.

MATERNAL AMINO ACIDS, PROTEINS, AND FETAL GROWTH AND DEVELOPMENT

TOTAL AMINO ACIDS

A striking relationship between maternal blood α-amino acid concentrations and birth weight, length, and cranial volume was observed in a prospective study of normal pregnant women at term (Table 8–3). Mothers with blood amino acid levels below 4 mg/100 ml had lighter and shorter babies with smaller cranial volumes than did those whose amino acid levels exceeded 4 mg/100 ml. No clear relationship between dietary intake as determined by recall and the blood amino acid levels was observed (30).

INDIVIDUAL AMINO ACIDS AND PROTEINS

In order to investigate the relationship of maternal blood amino acids and proteins to infant growth and mental development in human pregnancy, a prospective study was initiated in Detroit a few years ago. Eventually, 129 patients with uncomplicated pregnancies were enrolled (31). All were in social class V according to the Hollingshead–Redlich scale. Dietary assessments were made by estimating the amounts of nutrients ingested on 24-hour recall of food eaten.

Blood samples were obtained between weeks 32 and 34 (sample 1) and again between weeks 34 and 36 of gestation (sample 2) for determination of total levels of free α-amino acids and individual amino acids and for protein electrophoresis.

Table 8–3. MATERNAL BLOOD AMINO ACID LEVEL AND DEVELOPMENTAL MEASURES OF OFF-SPRING

| | **Mean** | | | | |
	Controls	Study group	No.	t	P
α-Amino acid					
N mg% blood	4.42	3.95	44	—	—
4.0 $\geq$ $\leq$ 3.9					
Birth weight (kg)	3.26	2.86	44	4.28	$<.001$
Spinal length					
Atlas to coccyx (mm)	208	196	42	3.6	$<.001$
Cranial capacity (cu cm)	453	421	43	2.73	$<.01$
Crown–heel length (mm)	483	460	42	2.70	$<.01$

Babies born from mothers with high amino acid levels in the last trimester were paired with those whose mothers had lower levels. They were matched for race, sex, and weeks of gestation at birth. C, control group; S, study group.

Birth weights and newborn lengths were recorded. Repeated cephalic measurements were made between 36 and 46 hours of life and were used to calculate the cranial volume. At 8 months (34 + 2 weeks) of age, each infant was evaluated by a psychologist using a standardized modification of the Bayley Scale of Infant Development.

Stepwise regression was employed to ascertain the amount of variance in birth weight, cranial volume, and infant mental (MDQ) and motor development (MOT) which could be explained by measures of maternal proteins, amino acids, and body dimensions. These maternal parameters served as independent variable predictors of infant mental and motor development.

Maternal factors such as prepregnancy weight, pregnancy weight gain, and height are shown in Table 8–4. Mean pregnancy weight gain was 12.2 + 6.7 kg, which is consistent with results obtained in other surveys (32). In Table 8–5, fetal measures and the result of Bayley infant mental and motor scales are recorded. Values obtained from the analysis of total and specific amino acids, total protein, and protein fractions in the first and second maternal blood sam-

Table 8–4. MATERNAL FACTORS (INDEPENDENT VARIABLES)*

Variables	Mean ± SD
Maternal height (cm)	161.3 ± 7.1
Prepregnancy weight (kg)	62.7 ± 15.7
Pregnancy weight gain (kg)	12.2 ± 6.7

*Moghissi KS, Churchill JA, Kurrie D: Am J Obstet Gynecol 123:398, 1975

Table 8–5. FETAL FACTORS (DEPENDENT VARIABLES)*

Variables	Mean ± SD
Birth weight (kg)	3.3 ± 0.5
Crown heel length (cm)	48.8 ± 2.9
Cranial volume (cu cm)	441.7 ± 57.6
Mental development (MDQ) (Score)	225.5 ± 16.1
Motor development (MOT) (Score)	35.3 ± 7.1

*Moghissi KS, Churchill JA, Kurrie D: Am J Obstet Gynecol 123:398, 1975

Table 8–6. MATERNAL PROTEINS IN THIRD TRIMESTER OF PREGNANCY (N = 129) (MEAN ± SD)*

Variables	Sample 1 (g/100 ml)	Sample 2 (g/100 ml)
Total protein	6.6 ± 0.5	6.7 ± 0.5
Albumin	3.5 ± 0.5	3.5 ± 0.4
Globulins	3.2 ± 0.4	3.3 ± 0.4
α_1-Globulin	0.4 ± 0.1	0.5 ± 0.2
α_2-Globulin	0.8 ± 0.2	0.8 ± 0.2
β-Globulin	1.0 ± 0.1	1.0 ± 0.2
γ-Globulin	1.0 ± 0.2	1.0 ± 0.3

*Moghissi KS, Churchill JA, Kurrie D: Am J Obstet Gynecol 123:398, 1975

ples (independent variables) are found in Tables 8–6 and 8–7. In Table 8–8 the intercorrelations among the four dependent variables of infants are reported. Birth weight is significantly related to cranial volume and motor development; whereas, mental development has no significant correlation with birth weight or cranial volume.

The four dependent variables in infants (birth weight, cranial volume, and the Bayley motor and mental scales) were correlated with 17 specific amino acid levels in sample 1 (Table 8–9) and sample 2 (Table 8–10). Fourteen of these 136 ($17 \times 4 \times 2 = 136$) correlations were significant, ten positively and four negatively, at or beyond the 5% level. At the 5% level of confidence, one would expect only seven correlations to be significant. With 14 correlations significant at the 5% level or beyond, there is clear evidence of a relationship between maternal amino acid level and fetal development. However, in sample 1 there were nine significant correlations out of 68, but in sample 2, only five. At the 5% level of confidence, we would expect four significant correlations. Thus for

Table 8–7. MATERNAL AMINO ACID LEVELS (MEAN ± SD)*

Variables	Sample 1 (mg/100 ml)	Sample 2 (mg/100 ml)
Total α-amino acid N	3.8 ± 0.4	4.0 ± 0.6
Lysine	1.5 ± 0.4	1.5 ± 0.4
Histidine	0.9 ± 0.2	1.0 ± 0.2
Ammonia	0.3 ± 0.2	0.4 ± 0.4
Arginine	0.4 ± 0.3	0.4 ± 0.3
Ornithine	0.4 ± 0.2	0.4 ± 0.2
Aspartic acid	1.3 ± 0.6	1.2 ± 0.5
Threonine	1.7 ± 0.4	1.7 ± 0.5
Serine	1.0 ± 0.3	1.0 ± 0.3
Proline	1.5 ± 0.6	1.7 ± 0.6
Glycine	1.2 ± 0.3	1.3 ± 0.4
Alanine	2.2 ± 0.5	2.3 ± 0.5
Valine	1.3 ± 0.4	1.3 ± 0.3
Isoleucine	0.5 ± 0.1	0.5 ± 0.1
Leucine	0.8 ± 0.2	0.9 ± 0.2
Tyrosine	0.6 ± 0.2	0.6 ± 0.1
Phenylalanine	0.6 ± 0.1	0.6 ± 0.1
Glutamine	0.6 ± 0.1	0.6 ± 0.1
Glutamic acid	0.7 ± 0.3	0.7 ± 0.3
Uric acid	4.2 ± 0.1	4.0 ± 0.6

*Moghissi KS, Churchill JA, Kurrie D: Am J Obstet Gynecol 123:398, 1975

Table 8–8. CORRELATION AMONG THE FOUR DEPENDENT VARIABLES (N = 129)‡

	Birth weight	Cranial volume	MOT	MDQ
Birth Weight (r)	1.00	0.703*	0.167†	0.004
Cranial Volume (r)		1.00	0.210†	0.079
MOT (r)			1.00	0.272*

MOT, motor development; MDQ, mental development.
*Significant at $P < 0.01$ using the 1-tailed t test.
†Significant at $P < 0.05$ using the 1-tailed t test.
‡Moghissi KS, Churchill JA, Kurrie D: Am J Obstet Gynecol 123:398, 1975

Table 8–9. CORRELATION OF DEPENDENT VARIABLES (BIRTH WEIGHT, CRANIAL VOLUME, MOTOR AND MENTAL DEVELOPMENT) WITH MATERNAL BLOOD AMINO ACIDS IN SAMPLE 1†

	Birth weight	Cranial volume	MOT	MDQ
Lysine (E)	0.06	0.06	−0.03	−0.13
Histidine (E)	0.07	0.15*	0.04	−0.05
Arginine (E)	0.01	0.07	−0.08	−0.05
Ornithine	0.06	0.05	0.05	−0.07
Aspartic acid	−0.07	−0.11	−0.04	−0.01
Threonine (E)	−0.05	−0.07	−0.07	−0.15
Serine	0.01	0.13	−0.07	0.00
Glutamic acid	−0.03	−0.16	−0.20*	−0.07
Proline	−0.06	0.01	−0.18*	−0.10
Glycine	0.16*	0.20*	0.15*	0.02
Alanine	−0.03	0.03	0.11	0.03
Valine (E)	−0.03	0.01	−0.05	0.07
Isoleucine (E)	0.04	0.17*	0.04	0.15*
Leucine (E)	0.03	0.11	0.04	0.12
Tyrosine	0.14	0.15*	0.05	0.01
Phenylalanine (E)	0.09	0.06	−0.02	0.02
Glutamine	−0.08	0.03	0.06	−0.13

E, essential amino acids; −, negative correlation.
*$P < 0.05$.
†Moghissi KS, Churchill JA, Kurrie D: Am J Obstet Gynecol 123:398, 1975

Table 8–10. CORRELATION OF DEPENDENT VARIABLES (BIRTH WEIGHT, CRANIAL VOLUME, MOTOR AND MENTAL DEVELOPMENT) WITH MATERNAL BLOOD AMINO ACIDS IN SAMPLE 2‡

	Birth weight	Cranial volume	MOT	MDQ
Lysine (E)	0.13	0.07	−0.08	−0.12
Histidine (E)	0.00	−0.03	0.09	−0.25*
Arginine (E)	−0.08	−0.09	−0.03	0.02
Ornithine	0.10	0.10	0.01	−0.18*
Aspartic acid	0.09	0.03	−0.02	−0.04
Threonine (E)	0.04	0.09	−0.11	−0.15
Serine	−0.02	0.03	−0.04	−0.13
Glutamic acid	0.10	0.13	0.03	−0.08
Proline	0.02	0.02	−0.10	−0.16
Glycine	0.10	0.25†	−0.06	−0.11
Alanine	−0.14	0.01	0.00	−0.11
Valine (E)	−0.12	−0.01	−0.07	0.05
Isoleucine (E)	−0.02	0.08	−0.06	0.03
Leucine (E)	−0.13	−0.02	−0.06	0.02
Tyrosine	−0.06	0.06	−0.01	0.10
Phenylalanine (E)	−0.08	0.05	0.01	0.05
Glutamine	−0.15*	0.23†	0.03	−0.10

E, essential amino acids; −, negative correlation.
*$P < 0.05$.
†$P < 0.005$.
‡Moghissi KS, Churchill JA, Kurrie D: Am J Obstet Gynecol 123:398, 1975

sample 1, twice as many correlations were significant at the 5% level or beyond than expected; whereas, for sample 2 only about the expected number were significant. This suggests that the effect of maternal amino acid level on fetal development may be more pronounced at 32 weeks (sample 1) than at 36 weeks (sample 2).

Similar correlations between the four dependent variables, maternal factors (prepregnancy weight, pregnancy weight gain, and height), total amino acid levels, and blood protein levels were effected (Tables 8–11 and 8–12). Maternal height, prepregnancy weight, weight gain during pregnancy, and maternal total amino acid levels were found to be significantly related to birth weight. Among proteins, only α_1-globulin showed significant correlation with cranial volume, MDQ, and MOT in sample 1, and with MDQ and MOT in sample 2.

Table 8–11. CORRELATION BETWEEN MATERNAL FACTORS (INDEPENDENT VARIABLES)§ AND EACH OF DEPENDENT VARIABLES IN SAMPLE 1

	Birth weight	Cranial volume	MOT	MDQ
Maternal height	0.28*	0.13	0.16†	0.10
Prepregnant weight	0.38*	0.26‡	−0.01	0.01
Weight gain (N=125)	0.18†	0.13	0.10	0.10
Amino acids	0.15†	0.07	0.10	0.05
Proteins	−0.02	−0.07	0.04	−0.04
Globulins	−0.03	−0.14	−0.01	−0.01
Albumin	−0.00	0.05	0.06	−0.02
α_1-Globulin	−0.10	−0.21‡	−0.22‡	−0.24‡
α_2-Globulin	0.00	−0.07	0.02	0.05
β-globulin	0.10	−0.04	−0.05	0.02
γ-globulin	−0.09	−0.11	0.09	0.08

−, Negative correlation.
*$P < 0.001$.
†$P < 0.05$.
‡$P < 0.01$.
§Moghissi KS, Churchill JA, Kurrie D: Am J Obstet Gynecol 123:398, 1975

Table 8–12. CORRELATION BETWEEN MATERNAL FACTORS (INDEPENDENT VARIABLES) AND EACH OF DEPENDENT VARIABLES‡ IN SAMPLE 2 (N = 129)

	Birth weight	Cranial volume	MOT	MDQ
Amino acids total	0.08	0.12	−0.00	0.09
Proteins total	0.01	−0.13	−0.12	−0.05
Globulins	0.02	−0.09	−0.07	−0.12
Albumin	−0.00	−0.04	−0.03	0.06
α_1-Globulin	0.04	−0.05	−0.18*	−0.21†
α_2-Globulin	−0.04	−0.07	−0.01	−0.01
β-Globulin	0.06	−0.11	−0.00	−0.06
γ-Globulin	−0.09	−0.07	−0.00	−0.05

−, Negative correlation.
*$P < 0.05$.
†$P < 0.01$.
‡Moghissi KS, Churchill JA, Kurrie D: Am J Obstet Gynecol 123:398, 1975

Three sets of stepwise regression analyses were run. Each set consisted of eight analyses (the four dependent variables by the two blood samples). The independent variables for the first set of regression analyses included only the 17 specific amino acid measures and the 5 protein fractions, i.e., albumin, α_1-, α_2-, β-, and γ-globulins. All of these analyses were significant at the 5% level or beyond (Tables 8–13 and 8–14). None of the 22 maternal blood measures from either sample 1 or 2 accounted for sufficient variance in birth weight to be selected by the analyses.

The mother's height and weight could reflect mechanisms (*e.g.,* hereditary) contributing to her amino acid and protein fraction levels as well as to fetal development independent of any direct effect of the former on the latter. Thus, a second set of regression analyses were run (Tables 8–15 and 8–16) which, in

Table 8–13. CONTRIBUTION (PERCENT VARIANCE) OF SIGNIFICANT MATERNAL BLOOD MEASURES TO THE FOUR DEPENDENT VARIABLES† (FIRST SET OF REGRESSION ANALYSIS) SAMPLE 1

	Percent of variance	P
Cranial volume		
α_1-Globulin*	4.6	0.01
Glycine	5.6	0.01
Together	10.2	0.01
Motor development		
α_1-Globulin*	4.9	0.05
Glycine	3.5	0.01
Proline*	2.9	0.05
All three	11.3	0.01
Mental development		
α_1-Globulin*	5.7	0.01
Glutamine*	3.0	0.01
Isoleucine	3.9	0.05
All three	12.6	0.01

*Negative correlation.
†Moghissi KS, Churchill JA, Kurrie D: Am J Obstet Gynecol 123:398, 1975

Table 8–14. CONTRIBUTION (PERCENT VARIANCE) OF SIGNIFICANT MATERNAL BLOOD MEASURES TO THE FOUR DEPENDENT VARIABLES† (FIRST SET OF REGRESSION ANALYSIS) SAMPLE 2

	Percent of variance	P
Cranial volume		
Glycine	6.3	0.01
Motor development		
α_1-Globulin*	4.6	0.05
Mental development		
α_1-Globulin*	3.3	0.05
Histidine*	6.5	0.01
Together	9.5	0.01

*Negative correlation.
†Moghissi KS, Churchill JA, Kurrie D: Am J Obstet Gynecol 123:398, 1975

addition to the 22 variables used in the first set, included also maternal height and prepregnant weight which were forced into the analyses prior to the stepwise inclusion of the 22 amino acid and protein fraction measures. These analyses show the significant contributions of the amino acid and protein fractions to four dependent developmental variables after maternal height and prepregnant weight have had the opportunity to account for their share of variability in the developmental variables. These analyses were also significant at the 5% level of confidence, or beyond (Tables 8–12 and 8–13). In the sample 1 analysis of birth weight, no amino acid or plasma fraction variables were selected. The third set of regression analyses differed from the second set only in that total amino acids, proteins, and globulins were also included.

Birth Weight

Maternal height and prepregnant weight accounted for about 16% in both the sample 1 and sample 2 analyses (Tables 8–15 and 8–16). Height was not significant in either case, but weight was significant for both variables. No maternal blood measures were selected from sample 1. In contrast, valine, lysine, and γ -globulins were selected from the sample 2 analysis. Thus, in sample 2, these

Table 8–15. CONTRIBUTION (PERCENT VARIANCE) OF MATERNAL HEIGHT AND WEIGHT AND SIGNIFICANT BLOOD MEASURES (SAMPLE 1) TO THE FOUR INFANT-DEPENDENT VARIABLES† (SECOND SET OF REGRESSION ANALYSIS)

	Percent of variance	P
Birth weight		
Maternal height	7.7	NS
Maternal weight (prepregnancy)	8.7	0.01
Total	16.4	0.01
Cranial volume		
Maternal height	1.6	NS
Maternal weight (prepregnancy)	5.0	0.05
α_1-Globulin*	4.6	0.01
Glycine	3.6	0.05
All together	14.8	0.01
Motor development		
Maternal height	2.5	NS
Maternal weight (prepregnancy)*	0.8	NS
α_1-Globulin*	4.7	0.01
Glycine	3.3	0.05
All together	11.3	0.01
Mental development		
Maternal height	1.2	NS
Maternal weight	0.1	NS
α_1-Globulin*	5.5	0.01
Glutamine*	3.0	0.01
Isoleucine	3.5	0.05
All together	13.1	0.01

NS, not significant.
*Negative correlation.
†Moghissi KS, Churchill JA, Kurrie D: Am J Obstet Gynecol 123:398, 1975

blood amino acid and protein measures accounted for an additional 11% of the variance in birth weight in the presence of the height and prepregnant weight in contrast to their behavior in the first part of analyses, suggesting that the relationships of some components of maternal valine, lysine, and γ-globulin in late pregnancy to infant birth weight may be quite independent of their relationship to maternal height and weight.

Only lysine, accounting for 4.6% of the variance in birth weight, had a positive correlation. The other two blood factors were negatively correlated. When total amino acids and proteins were included in the regression analysis, similar results were obtained for sample 2. For sample 1, total amino acids, threonine (negative correlation), and glycine were also selected and contributed an additional 9% to the birth weight.

Cranial Volume

Maternal height was not significantly correlated with cranial volume, but prepregnant weight was significant for both samples 1 and 2 analyses (5% of the variance). Other blood measures which contributed significantly to cranial volume were glycine (which appeared in all analyses of sample 1), glutamine

Table 8–16. CONTRIBUTION (PERCENT VARIANCE) OF MATERNAL HEIGHT AND WEIGHT AND SIGNIFICANT BLOOD MEASURES (SAMPLE 2) TO THE FOUR INFANT DEPENDENT VARIABLES† (SECOND SET OF REGRESSION ANALYSIS)

	Percent of variance	P
Birth weight		
Maternal height	7.6	NS
Maternal weight (prepregnancy)	8.7	0.01
Valine*	3.1	0.01
Lysine	4.6	0.01
γ-Globulin*	3.3	0.05
All together	27.3	0.01
Cranial volume		
Maternal height	1.6	NS
Maternal weight (prepregnancy)	5.3	0.01
Glutamine	4.6	0.05
β-globulin*	3.4	0.05
Total	17.0	0.01
Motor development		
Maternal height	2.4	NS
Maternal weight (prepregnancy)*	0.8	NS
α_1-Globulin*	4.2	0.05
All together	7.4	0.05
Mental development		
Maternal height	1.1	NS
Maternal weight	0.1	NS
Histidine*	7.4	0.01
α_1-Globulin*	3.2	0.05
All together	11.8	0.01

*Negative correlation.
NS, not significant.
†Moghissi KS, Churchill JA, Kurrie D: Am J Obstet Gynecol 123:398, 1975

(positively), glutamic acid, threonine, histidine, and α_1- and β-globulins (negatively). Maternal blood variables selected accounted for no more—or even less —of the variance in birth weight and cranial volume than did prepregnant weight.

Motor Development

Maternal height and weight accounted for about 3% of the variance in both samples 1 and 2 analyses (Tables 8–15 and 8–16). However, neither was statistically significant. α_1-Globulin, again, made a consistent appearance, correlating negatively with motor development. Glycine was the only amino acid which contributed to motor development (Tables 8–10 and 8–12).

Mental Development

Maternal height and weight made no significant contribution to mental development. Histidine and α_1-globulin (both negatively correlated) accounted for 9.5–11% of the variance in mental development for the sample 2 analysis. For the sample 1 analysis, α_1-globulin, glutamine, and isoleucine were selected and accounted for about 12% of the variance.

It is evident that the infant developmental variables studied are not independent of the maternal blood protein and amino acid measures, even in the presence of maternal height and prepregnant weight contributions.

Maternal blood measures tend also to contribute more than maternal height and prepregnancy weight to motor and mental developments. In contrast, maternal amino acids and proteins seem to account for about the same amount, or appreciably less, of the variability in birth weight and cranial volume as does maternal prepregnant weight. α_1-Globulin was the only variable selected by all sets of analyses and for all samples in the motor and mental development analyses.

COMMENT

The above studies indicate that the level of certain maternal amino acids and proteins correlate significantly with fetal growth and development.

The observation that prepregnancy weight and pregnancy weight gain contribute significantly to the birth weight has been previously reported and is confirmed in this study. On the contrary, despite some published reports, maternal height showed no significant correlation with infant developmental measures (34, 41). Prepregnancy weight and maternal weight gain during pregnancy in the absence of complications such as toxemia may be considered as indirect evidence of the maternal nutritional state. Pregnancy weight gain is a result of protein and fat accumulation, and salt and water retention together with the weight of the product of conception. Fetal nutrition may result not only from nutrients ingested by the mother during pregnancy but also from maternal reserve (prepregnancy status) when they are needed. In fact, Habicht *et al.* (18) have reported that chronic limitation of calories during pregnancy is associated with lowered birth weight and that supplementary feeding offered to pregnant women (in rural Guatemalan villages) caused a rise of mean birth weight in their offspring. The positive association between maternal caloric ingestion from food supplement and birth weight was observed whether the calories were ingested early or late in pregnancy.

In addition to these maternal factors, amino acids (particularly lysine, valine, and probably, glycine and threonine) are significantly related to birth weight. Lysine is well known for its profound effect on animal growth.

Cranial volume seems to be related less to maternal prepregnant weight than amino acid and protein measures. Glycine, glutamine, α_1-globulin, β-globulin, glutamic acid, threonine, histidine, tyrosine, and isoleucine all appeared to correlate with cranial volume, but glycine contributed most significantly, independent of maternal height and prepregnancy weight. α_1-Globulin, β-globulin, threonine, histidine, and glutamic acid all negatively correlated with cranial volume.

The contribution of maternal height and prepregnant weight to motor development was small. It was insignificant so far as mental development was concerned. α_1-Globulin and glycine contributed most to motor development. α_1-Globulin, glutamic acid, and proline correlated negatively with motor development. Therefore, the rise of α_1-globulin, glutamic acid, and proline levels in late pregnancy may have some predictive value on diminished motor development of the infant. Also, elevation of α_1-globulin, glutamine, and histidine levels and depression of isoleucine levels may be indicative of lowered mental development.

These data suggest that specific proteins or amino acids may be responsible for different developmental measures. Certain amino acids and proteins appear to contribute to physical growth, whereas, others are related to infant mental or motor development.

The consistent negative correlation of α_1-globulin with several developmental measures is interesting. Major proteins migrating electrophoretically in α_1-zone include α_1-lipoprotein (concerned with the transport of lipids, hormones, and fat-soluble vitamins), orosomucoid, α_1-antitrypsin, α_1-glycoprotein, transcortin, and thyroxin-binding globulin. Negative contribution of α_1-globulin to infant motor and particularly mental development may result from abnormal increase of any one of these protein fractions. Studies are required to clarify further this point. Histidine in sample 2 was also found to contribute negatively in a consistent manner to mental development. Histidine has been extensively studied in pregnancy and is found in large amount in the urine of parturients (29). It is also known that in histidinemia, a genetic disorder, the elevated blood level of histidine in the infant is associated with mental retardation (9).

No babies with congenital malformation were born in these studies. Thus, genetic and other embryonal impairments did not interfere with fetal development. However, some babies with intrauterine growth retardation caused by uteroplacental insufficiency were probably intermingled with those whose dysmaturity was considered to be due to intrauterine malnutrition. Their presence in an unknown proportion in the data pool might reduce to some extent the positive correlation between maternal chemicals and infant developmental variables. Hypothetically, placental insufficiency may prevent normal or even elevated levels of maternal amino acids and proteins to reach the fetus; whereas, in malnourished women, the fetal stunting is related to depressed maternal protein and amino acid measures. It is interesting that despite strict control of socioeconomic status, which also limits the range of nutritional variation, the data reported here resulted in statistically significant findings.

PRACTICAL CONSIDERATIONS

Based on the results of these studies, certain practical considerations are in order. There is evidence that maternal nutritional status before and during pregnancy influence fetal birth weight and brain development. Therefore, excessive dietary restrictions in pregnancy are ill advised. The lack of certain amino acids in the diet of pregnant women may have deleterious effect. Furthermore, the quality of ingested food during gestation may exert important effects on functional ability of the brain in later life.

The data reported here also suggest that the determination of levels of α_1-globulin and a few amino acids such as glycine, lysine, and histidine in late pregnancy may be used as possible predictors of fetal growth and development.

Amino acids reach the fetus by systemic transport through the placenta or by ingestion of the amniotic fluid. Similarly, certain proteins cross the placental barrier, and most of those found in the amniotic fluid are swallowed and used for fetal nutrition.

Intrauterine fetal malnutrition may result from inadequate maternal dietary intake or reserve (prepregnancy nutritional status), malabsorption, metabolic disorders associated with liver and kidney disease, or impairment of placental function resulting from inadequate blood flow.

It is reasonable to assume that the nutritional condition of the fetus may be improved by intravenous or intraamniotic infusion of amino acids and/or proteins. Several preliminary studies dealing with intraamniotic infusion of amino acids have recently been published.

Renaud et al. (36) injected a mixture of amino acids into the amniotic cavity of normal pregnant women and those with a variety of obstetric conditions such as toxemia of pregnancy, premature labor, and intrauterine fetal growth retardation. They found that immediately after injection the concentration of amniotic fluid amino acids rose. One hour after the injection amniotic fluid, amino acid levels had considerably decreased and between one-third to two-thirds of the injected amino acids had left the amniotic cavity. After 48 hours, amniotic fluid amino acids had reached normal levels. A selective study of individual amino acids in the amniotic fluid 45 minutes after intraamniotic injection revealed that the percentage of disappearance was not the same for all amino acids. The amino acids which disappeared most rapidly consisted of asparate–asparagine, lysine, 86%; methionine, 82%; isoleucine, 81%; leucine, 74%; alanine, 74%; phenylalanine, 73%; tyrosine, 73%; and threonine, 70%. The maternal venous aminoacidogram was not altered. The authors were unable to demonstrate an increase in the concentrations of amino acids of the umbilical blood (samples obtained 85 hours after injection) and hypothesized that the amino acids could have been stored or rapidly metabolized by the fetus. The placenta very rapidly took up a considerable proportion of the injected amino acids and showed a significant increase in its content of all amino acids but cystine and ornithine. Repeated intraamniotic injection did not appear to have an adverse effect on the fetus and the neonate. In certain cases of intrauterine growth retardation, a return of maternal urinary estriol to normal ranges was observed.

These studies clearly show that amino acids injected into the amniotic fluid reach the fetus and may be utilized for the synthesis of proteins.

Since specific amino acids may be responsible for different developmental measures, an excessive concentration of certain amino acids may have deleterious effect. The selection of amino acids for intraamniotic infusion is therefore of critical importance. Whether or not the gastrointestinal tract of the fetus is capable of selecting from ingested and hyrolyzed proteins or amino acids those which are beneficial to its growth and development while rejecting those which may be harmful remains to be elucidated.

REFERENCES

1. Beckman G, Von Schoultz B, Stigbrand T: The "pregnancy zone" protein and fetal welfare. Acta Obstet Gynecol Scand 53:59, 1974
2. Brasel J, Winick M: Regulation of nucleic acid synthesis in fetus and placenta during normal growth and maturation. In Moghissi KS (ed): Birth Defects and Fetal Development, Endocrine and Metabolic Factors. Springfield, Ill, CC Thomas, 1974, p 5
3. Caldwell DF, Churchill JA: Learning ability in the progeny of rats administered a protein deficient diet during the second half of gestation. Neurology (Minneap) 17:95, 1967
4. Clarke HCM, Freeman T, Pryse–Phillips W: Serum proteins in normal pregnancy and mild pre-eclampsia. J Obstet Gynaecol Br Commonw 78:105, 1971
5. Dallaire L, Potier M, Melancon SB, Patrick J: Feto-maternal amino acid metabolism. J Obstet Gynaecol Br Commonw 81:761, 1974
6. Dobbing J: The influence of early nutrition on the development of myelination of the brain. Proc R Soc Lond [Biol] 159:503, 1964
7. Dobbing J: Effects of experimental undernutrition on development of the nervous system. In Scrimshaw NS, Gordon JE (eds): Malnutrition, Learning, and Behavior. Cambridge, MIT Press, 1968, pp 181–202
8. Fischbacher PH, Quinlivan WL: Qualitative and quantitative analysis of the proteins in human amniotic fluid. Am J Obstet Gynecol 108:1051, 1970
9. Ghadimi H, Partington MB, Hunter A: A familial disturbance of histidine metabolism. N Engl J Med 265:221, 1961
10. Ghadimi H, Pecora P: Free amino acids of cord plasma as compared with maternal plasma during pregnancy. Pediatrics 33:500, 1964
11. Glendening MB, Margolis AJ, Page EW: Amino acid concentrations in fetal and maternal plasma. Am J Obstet Gynecol 81:591, 1961
12. Gitlin D: Protein transport across the placenta and protein turnover between amni-

otic fluid, maternal and fetal circulations. In Moghissi KS, Hafez ESE (eds): The Placenta: Biological and Clinical Aspects. Springfield, Ill, CC Thomas, 1974, pp 151–191

13. Gitlin D, Biasucci A: Development of γG, γA, γM, β1C/ β1A, C'1 esterase inhibitor, ceruloplasmin, transferrin, hemopexin, haptoglobin, fibrinogen, plasminogen, α_1-antitrypsin, orosomucoid, β-lipoprotein, α_2-macroglobulin and prealbumin in the human conceptus. J Clin Invest 48:1433, 1969

14. Gitlin D, Biasucci A: Ontogenesis of immunoreactive growth hormone, follicle-stimulating hormone, thyroid-stimulating hormone, luteinizing hormone, chorionic prolactin and chorionic gonadotropin in the human conceptus. J Clin Endocrinol Metab 29:926, 1969

15. Gitlin D, Kumate J, Morales C, Noriega L, Arevalo N: The turnover of amniotic fluid protein in the human conceptus. Am J Obstet Gynecol 113:632, 1972

16. Gitlin D, Kumate J, Urrusti J, Morales C: The selectivity of the human placenta in the transfer of plasma proteins from mother to fetus. J Clin Invest 43:1938, 1964

17. Gitlin D, Kumate J, Urrusti J, Morales C: Selective and directional transfer of 7S γ $_2$-globulin across the human placenta. Nature 203:86, 1964

18. Habicht JP, Yarbrough C, Lechtig A, Klein RE: Relation of maternal supplementary feeding during pregnancy to birth weight and other sociobiological factors. In Winick M (ed): Nutrition and Fetal Development, Vol 2. New York, John Wiley & Son, 1974, p 127

19. Holley WL, Churchill JA: Physical and mental deficits of twinning. In Perinatal Factors Affecting Human Development. Washington DC, Scientific publication No. 185, Pan American Health Organization, 1969, p 24

20. Holley WL, Rosenbaum AL, Churchill JA: Effect of rapid succession of pregnancy. In Perinatal Factors Affecting Human Development. Washington DC, Scientific publication No. 185, Pan American Health Organization, 1969, p 41

21. Johnson AM, Umansky I, Alper CA, Everett C, Greenspan G: Amniotic fluid proteins: maternal and fetal contributions. J Pediatr 84:588, 1974

22. Johnstone FD, MacGillivray I, Dennis KJ: Nitrogen retention in pregnancy. J Obstet Gynaecol Br Commonw 79:777, 1972

23. Lev R, Orlic D: Uptake of protein in swallowed amniotic fluid by monkey fetal intestine in utero. Gastroenterology 65:60, 1973

24. Levy HL, Montag P: Free amino acids in human amniotic fluid. A quantitative study by ion-exchange chromatography. Pediatr Res 3:113, 1969

25. Lindblad BS, Baldestan A: The normal venous plasma free amino-acid levels of non-pregnant women and of mother and child during delivery. Acta Paediatr Scand 56:37, 1967

26. Mack HC: The plasma proteins. Clin Obstet Gynecol 3:336, 1960

27. Mandelbaum B, Evans TN: Life in the amniotic fluid. Am J Obstet Gynecol 104:365, 1969

28. Metcoff J: Biochemical markers of intrauterine malnutrition. In Winick M (ed): Nutrition and Fetal Development, Vol 2. New York, John Wiley & Sons, 1974, p 27

29. Moghissi KS: Métabolisme des acides aminés pendant la grossesse et son appréciation par la chromatographie sur papier. Geneva, Thesis Édition Médicine et Hygiéne, 1951

30. Moghissi KS, Churchill JA, Frohman C: Relationship of maternal amino acid blood levels to fetal development. In Perinatal Factors Affecting Human Development. Washington DC, Scientific publication No. 185, Pan American Health Organization, 1969, p 16

31. Moghissi KS, Churchill JA, Kurrie D: Relationship of maternal amino acids and proteins to fetal growth and mental development. Am J Obstet Gynecol 123:398, 1975

32. Oakes GK, Chez RA: Nutrition during pregnancy. Contemporary Obstet Gynecol 4:147, 1974

33. Osofsky HJ: Antenatal malnutrition: its relationship to subsequent infant and child development. Am J Obstet Gynecol 105:1150, 1969
34. Ounsted M: Familial factors affecting fetal growth. In Perinatal Factors Affecting Human Development. Washington DC, Scientific publication No. 185, Pan American Health Organization, 1965, p 60
35. Reid DWJ, Campbell DJ, Yakymyshyn LY: Quantitative amino acids in amniotic fluid and maternal plasma in early and late pregnancy. Am J Obstet Gynecol 111:251, 1971
36. Renaud R, Kirschtetter L, Koehl C, Boog G, Brettes JP, Schumacher JC, Vincendon G, Willard D, Gandar R: Amino-acid intra-amniotic injections. In Persianinov LS, Chervakova TV, Presl J (eds): Recent Progress in Obstetrics and Gynaecology. Amsterdam, Excerpta Medica, 1974, pp 234–256
37. Saling E, Dudenhausen JW, Kynast G: Basic investigations about intra-amniotic compensatory nutrition of the malnourished fetus. In Persianinov LS, Chervakova TV, Presl J (eds): Recent Progress in Obstetrics and Gynaecology. Amsterdam, Excerpta Medica, 1974, pp 227–233
38. Schoultz von BO: A quantitative study of the pregnancy zone protein in the sera of pregnant and puerperal women. Am J Obstet Gynecol 119:792, 1974
39. Seppala M, Ruoslahti E: Alpha fetoprotein in maternal serum: a new marker for detection of fetal distress and intrauterine death. Am J Obstet Gynecol 115:48, 1973
40. Sowards DL, Monif GRG: Serum immunoglobulin M levels between weeks 22 and 37 of gestation. Am J Obstet Gynecol 112:394, 1972
41. Weiss W, Jackson EC: Maternal factors affecting birth weight. In Perinatal Factors Affecting Human Development. Washington DC, Scientific publication No. 185, Pan American Health Organization, 1965, p 54
42. Winick M: Cellular growth in intrauterine malnutrition. Pediatr Clin North Am 17:69, 1970
43. Young M, Prenton MA: Maternal and fetal plasma amino acid concentrations during gestation and in retarded fetal growth. J Obstet Gynaecol Br Commonw 76:333, 1969
44. Zamenof S, VanMarthens E, Grauel L: Prenatal cerebral development: effect of restricted diet, reversal by growth hormone. Science 174:954, 1971
45. Zinneman HH, Seal US, Doe R: Urinary amino acids in pregnancy, following progesterone, and estrogen-progesterone. J Clin Endocrinol Metab 27:397, 1967
46. Zuspan FP, Goodrich S: Metabolic studies in normal pregnancy. I. Nitrogen metabolism. Am J Obstet Gynecol 100:7, 1968

Chapter 9

The Effect of Maternal Alcohol Ingestion During Pregnancy on Offspring

Eileen M. Ouellette, Henry L. Rosett

Alcohol, our most widely used drug, may be a major cause of fetal malformations. Excessive alcohol ingestion has long been known to damage the mature nervous system. Despite the historical notation of alcohol as a possible direct toxin to the fetus, the modern view has been that alcohol places the child at risk more in a social and psychologic sense than a direct physical sense. Recently, attention has been directed to the possible teratogenic effects on offspring of chronic maternal alcohol ingestion during pregnancy, the features of which have been grouped under the term *fetal alcohol syndrome.*

DRINKING AMONG AMERICAN WOMEN

According to the most recent report of the National Institute of Alcoholism and Alcohol Abuse to the United States Congress, the proportion of women in the United States who drink heavily is increasing rapidly. The age group from 21 to 29 appears to have the highest proportion of heavy drinkers (23).

Estimates of the ratio of female to male alcoholics range from 1:5 to 1:1. The total population of alcoholics in the United States is estimated to be 9 million, and there may be between 1.5–4.5 million female alcoholics. With changing attitudes toward women drinking and the increased availability of alcoholism treatment programs, more heavy drinkers are being discovered among young females. Belfer *et al.* (1) stress that alcoholic women have been a largely unknown group in terms of number, psychologic characteristics, and the nature of their drinking patterns. These investigators found that, in 20 of 34 alcoholic women, drinking increased during the premenstrual period. It is very likely that the physiologic changes of pregnancy and the psychologic stress from the demands of motherhood could be additional factors leading to alcoholism.

The increase in alcohol consumption by women during the childbearing years has renewed attention to the possible relationship between alcohol consumption, faulty infant development, and the fetal alcohol syndrome. Maternal alcohol consumption may contribute to physical abnormalities at birth and in early life and to inadequate mothering practices which subsequently retard the growth and development of infants.

MATERNAL DRINKING AND FETAL ABNORMALITIES

HISTORICAL REVIEW

Anecdotes concerning the presumed ill effects of parental alcohol ingestion date to antiquity. Both Carthage and Sparta had laws prohibiting alcohol use by newly married couples to prevent conception while intoxicated. Aristotle noted that "foolish, drunken or harebrained women most often bring forth children like unto themselves, morose and languid" (2).

Subsequently, in the eighteenth and nineteenth centuries, substantial literature developed on the harm of maternal alcoholism on children. In England from 1720 to 1750, traditional restrictions on grain distilling were lifted, and the so-called gin epidemic swept the country. A plethora of warnings were published. In 1726, the College of Physicians petitioned Parliament for control of the distilling trade, citing gin as "a cause of weak, feeble and distempered children" (8). In 1834, a select committee of the House of Commons investigating drunkenness indicated that infants born to alcoholic mothers sometimes had a "starved, shriveled and imperfect look" (35).

By the midnineteenth century, reports of abnormalities in offspring of alcoholics began to appear in America. In 1857, Stevens warned that the offspring of such parents inherited "a weak and perverted nervous system overthrown by the least unusual exciting cause, subject to spasms, convulsions, and falling readily into attacks of epilepsy or idiocy" (38). During the late nineteenth and early twentieth centuries, numerous reports in France, Germany, and England cited an increased frequency of abortions, stillbirths, neonatal deaths, retardation of growth and development, epilepsy, and other neurologic disorders in such offspring (4, 16, 44).

Grouping the adverse effects of parental alcoholism without separating paternal from maternal influences, together with a persisting interest in the deleterious influence of acute alcoholic intoxication at the time of conception led to a gradual discreditation of these theories (4, 9). With the advent of prohibition in the United States in 1919, a dramatic decrease in medical articles concerning alcohol and pregnancy occurred, and speculation concerning the teratogenic effects of alcohol disappeared from the English and American medical literature.

MODERN CLINICAL STUDIES

In the French literature, however, reports of a higher incidence of retardation and neurologic disorders in offspring of alcoholics continued to appear (4, 9). In 1951, Desclaux and Morton (4) reported a large group of retarded children of alcoholics with epilepsy and electroencephalographic abnormalities. Rouquette (9) described 100 offspring of alcoholics in whom a high incidence of low birth weight was found and in whom retardation of postnatal growth in height and weight occurred. In 1968, Lemoine et al. (20) reported for the first time a characteristic appearance among 127 offspring of alcoholic mothers:

short stature and diminished weight, a peculiar facies, and psychomotor retardation.

In 1972, Ulleland (45) reviewed newborn nursery and delivery records to identify all undergrown infants born in an 18-month period. Personnel of the prenatal clinic were asked to identify, retrospectively, known alcoholics and any women who were intoxicated when seen in the clinic. Eighty-three percent of the infants born to the alcoholic mothers were small for gestational age, compared with 2.3% of the infants of nonalcoholic mothers.

Jones *et al.* (19), in 1973, described for the first time in the United States a recognizable pattern of multiple congenital anomalies with microcephaly, micrognathia, microphthalmia, cardiac defects, prenatal and postnatal growth retardation, and developmental delay in 8 children born to unrelated alcoholic mothers. A few months later, 3 additional cases of this disorder were described by Jones and his associates. The term fetal alcohol syndrome is applied to this constellation of growth and other morphologic abnormalities found among offspring of alcoholic women.

Jones and colleagues (17, 18) reviewed charts from the National Institute of Neurological Diseases and Stroke (NINDS) study of 55,000 pregnancies. Direct questions about alcohol use had not been included when the original data were gathered. The NINDS staff noted gross clinical evidence of maternal alcoholism in 69 charts. Thirty-five of these records had sufficient historical and pathophysiologic data to meet the National Council on Alcoholism's criteria for alcoholism (6). Twenty-three of the 35 mothers continued to drink heavily throughout pregnancy, while 12 reported that they stopped drinking while pregnant. These 23 cases were compared with a matched control group. Four of the 23 infants born to these mothers died during the perinatal period. The mortality rate of 17% contrasted with a 2% mortality rate in the matched control group. Thirty-two percent of the 23 children showed evidence of the fetal alcohol syndrome, while only 1 child born to one of the 12 mothers who stopped drinking while pregnant had signs of the syndrome.

In 1974, we reported familial cases of the fetal alcohol syndrome. Three pregnancies in an alcoholic woman, each by a different father, resulted in offspring with multiple minor congenital anomalies, microcephaly, and developmental delay (28). Since that time we have reported an additional family of three such children, each also fathered by different men (27). In each of two families with 3 children with the fetal alcohol syndrome, each successive child has been more significantly impaired.

To date, autopsy material is available in only 1 recognized human case of the fetal alcohol syndrome (4). This infant died at age 5 days and had a brain weight of 140 g (normal, 400 g) (50). The brain showed lissencephaly (or a smooth appearance), lacked the normal gyration and sulcation pattern, and resembled a fetal brain during the second to fourth gestational months (3, 21). Agenesis of the corpus callosum, which occurs between the first to fourth gestational months, was also present.

PROSPECTIVE STUDY AT THE BOSTON CITY HOSPITAL

Little is known about the frequency and spectrum of the fetal alcohol syndrome. Issues such as the quantity, frequency, and variability of alcohol consumption before conception and during the various phases of pregnancy have not yet been examined systematically. It can be hypothesized that heavy drinking during the first trimester may have the greatest effect on fetal maldevelopment, while heavy alcohol consumption near term may affect nutrition and delivery.

Obviously, not all offspring of alcoholic women are abnormal. If maternal alcohol ingestion during pregnancy is teratogenic to the fetus, many instances of previously unexplained congenital anomalies, especially microcephaly and developmental delay, may be understood.

A pilot prospective study was set up at the Boston City Hospital to study some of these issues. Beginning in May 1974, a random sample of women registering for prenatal care for the first time at the Boston City Hospital were interviewed using a structured interview questionnaire. The interview determined the volume and variability of maternal alcohol intake, as well as the use of other drugs, smoking, and nutritional status. Demographic data also were obtained. Drinking patterns were classified using Cahalan's Volume-Variability Index, which entails a two-step operation (3). Each woman was classified according to her average daily volume, and these groups were divided into subgroups according to how much the woman's alcohol intake varied from day to day. Separate inquiry was made about the use of wine, beer, and liquor. The monthly volume of alcohol was calculated by multiplying frequency of use of each beverage by the various quantities usually consumed. Division by 30 yielded the daily volume. Variability was established as either high-maximum (5 or more drinks) or low-maximum (fewer than 5 drinks). Women who drank less than once a month were classified as abstinent or rare drinkers; women who drank (at least once a month) up to 2.2 ounces of absolute alcohol daily were defined as moderate drinkers, and were further subdivided according to their average daily volume. Heavy drinkers consumed between 2.3 and 15 ounces of absolute alcohol per day, with a mean of 5.9 ounces.

At the time of delivery, the infants were given detailed pediatric, neurologic, and developmental examinations without prior knowledge of the history of the mother or baby. Additional information concerning pregnancy and delivery history was obtained, but only following coding of the data obtained on the physical examination.

RESULTS

To date, 305 women with a mean age of 23½ years have participated in the study. Fifty-three percent are married or living with the father of the baby; 47% have never been married or are separated or divorced. Their ethnic composition reflects that of the inner city area served by the Boston City Hospital: 52% black, 29% white, 14% Hispanic, and 5% American Indian and Oriental. They are a relatively poor population, with 66% estimating their monthly income under $500.00. Forty-seven percent of these women are primigravidas.

Only 10% of the entire population met the recommended dietary allowance of the National Research Council for at least seven of the nine nutrient categories. In all groups the women's diet contained excess starches and few fresh fruits or vegetables. There was no significant difference in nutrition among drinking and nondrinking women, and none were considered seriously malnourished.

Forty-three percent of the women smoked. Twelve percent stopped smoking with the onset of pregnancy, and 34% abstained from both alcohol and cigarettes. Of the heavy drinkers who also smoked, 78% consumed a package or more of cigarettes per day. Heavy drinking women tended to smoke more than nondrinking women, although 20% of the heavy drinkers did not smoke at all.

Of the 302 women studied, 144 women or 48% were abstinent or rare drinkers; 136 or 45% drank moderately, and 22 or 7% were heavy drinkers. Many of the heavy drinking women reported that they had reduced their alcohol consumption to some extent during this pregnancy. When data on the rare, moderate, and heavy drinkers were compared, no significant differences were found in age, race, religion, income, or nutrition.

Use of psychoactive drugs other than alcohol was reported by less than 10% of our patients. Pregnant heroin addicts, however, are referred to a special methadone maintenance program and are not represented in this study.

Of the 134 babies born to date, 54 or 40% have been born to rarely drinking or abstinent mothers, 65 or 49% to moderate drinkers, and 15 or 11% to heavy drinking women. There have been two therapeutic abortions and no stillbirths or neonatal deaths. Comparing the results of examinations on the offspring of mothers in all drinking groups, no differences were found in 1-minute and 5-minute Apgar scores, nor was there any difference in the frequency of acquired medical illness.

Infants were classified as abnormal if congenital anomalies were present or if the infants showed growth abnormalities, were jittery, or displayed abnormalities of tone. Only 4 of 15 infants born to heavy drinking women or 27% were considered to be normal at the time of the newborn examination, compared with 54% in the moderate drinking group and 60% in the abstinent group. The population at Boston City Hospital is a high-risk group, with 35% of all newborns delivered there admitted to the intensive care unit, which may account for the large number of abnormal infants in the abstinent and moderate drinking groups (Fig. 9-1).

A surprising number of babies in all groups showed hypotonia and/or jitteriness, but again, those signs were more frequent with increasing maternal alcohol intake. Single, minor congenital anomalies were found in all three groups. Only 1 child of the 54 born to mothers in the lowest drinking group had a major anomaly, as did 1 child of the 65 born to moderate drinkers. Congenital anomalies were present in 5 of the 15 babies born to heavy drinking women. Two infants were microcephalic, and 2 had polydactyly. A transverse palmar crease, a minor anomaly, was present in an additional child. One child with microcephaly also displayed a beaked nose, micrognathia, and redundant skin on the neck.

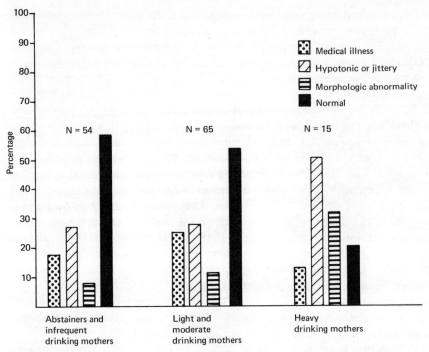

Fig. 9–1. Frequency of abnormality in newborn infants of drinking mothers.

Fig. 9–2. Frequency of growth abnormalities in newborn infants of drinking mothers.

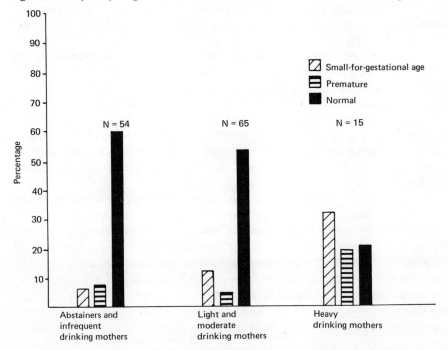

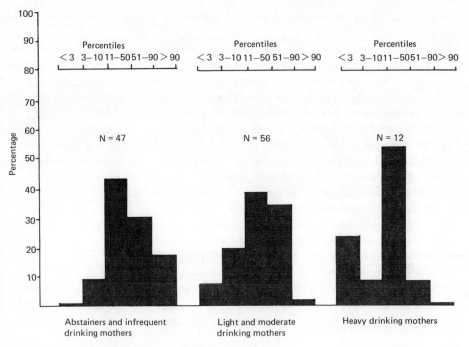

Fig. 9–3. Birth length in infants of drinking mothers.

Fig. 9–4. Birth weight in infants of drinking mothers.

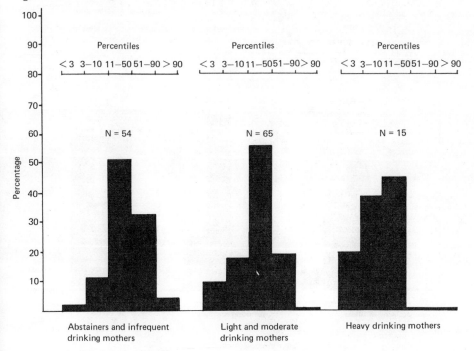

Except for 2 cases of microcephaly, no consistent pattern of anomalies was noted.

When growth parameters were compared, the frequency of prematurity differed among the three drinking groups: 7% in the abstinent group, 4% in the moderate group, and 20% in the heavy drinking group. A marked increase in infants found to be small for gestational age was noted with increased alcohol intake, ranging from 5% in infants born to mothers in the abstinent group, to 12% in the moderate group, to 33% in the heavy drinking group (Fig. 9–2).

Major differences were found in growth parameters among the three groups of babies. Birth length was distributed throughout all percentiles among the infants of abstainers and moderate drinkers but was clustered at the lower percentiles among offspring of heavy drinking women. Only 1 child born to a heavy drinker was above the 50th percentile for length (Fig. 9–3).

A similar trend was found when birth weights were compared. No child whose weight was above the 50th percentile was born to a heavy drinking mother, and 3 of 15 or 20% were below the 3rd percentile (Fig. 9–4).

Smaller head circumferences were found more frequently among the offspring of heavy drinking women than in the offspring of the abstinent or moderate drinking groups. No child born to a heavy drinking mother was found to have a head circumference above the 50th percentile, and 2 were microcephalic (Fig. 9–5).

Fig. 9–5. Head circumference in infants of drinking mothers.

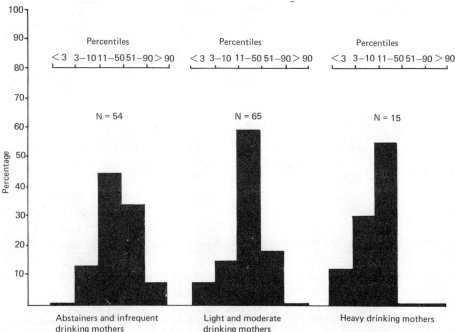

OTHER POSSIBLE TERATOGENIC FACTORS

At the present time, very little more is known about the spectrum of the fetal alcohol syndrome. Issues such as the quantity, frequency, and variability of alcohol consumption before conception and during the various stages of pregnancy have not yet been examined systematically. It can be hypothesized that heavy drinking during the first trimester may have the greatest effect on fetal development, while heavy alcohol consumption near term may affect nutrition and the obstetrical delivery. Continued maternal alcohol consumption during the neonatal period may contribute to child neglect, failure to thrive, and child abuse.

The firm establishment of the teratogenic role of alcohol in the production of these anomalies is critical in view of the fact that malnutrition and vitamin deficiency (particularly of thiamine and folic acid), smoking and drug abuse, hypoglycemia, and deficiency of trace metals may be proposed as alternative etiologic factors. The latter possibilities suggest that there may be a specific intervention or series of interventions which can prevent the syndrome.

Malnutrition

A voluminous literature, from both clinical and experimental studies, has evolved from the study of malnutrition (5, 22, 37, 39, 40, 47–49). Smith studied the effects of acute severe malnutrition on pregnancy in several hundred pregnant women in Holland during the final days of World War II (37). This work demonstrated an increase in small and premature infants, but malformed infants accounted for only 0.5% of the deliveries. More recent work among the poorer people in Latin America demonstrated diminished stature, head size, and intellectual accomplishments in offspring of chronically malnourished mothers, but an increased occurrence of malformations was not noted (5). Stoch and Smythe (39, 40) in South Africa also found that malnutrition in early life impaired body growth, especially body weight, to a greater extent than head growth and psychomotor development. If such children are fed suitable diets postnatally, catch-up growth occurs (22).

By contrast, in infants with the fetal alcohol syndrome, the head circumference and body length are affected more than body weight, and this discrepancy persists postnatally even with an adequate diet. In addition, many mothers of patients with the fetal alcohol syndrome have been carefully followed throughout their pregnancies, and malnutrition has not been noted (4, 19, 28). The present study demonstrated a statistically significant decrease in all growth parameters and in the frequency of congenital malformations in infants of mothers with excessive alcohol intake. There are no significant differences in nutritional intake among all groups in our population to account for these findings.

Vitamin Deficiency

Blood levels of vitamins A and C and folic acid have been measured in several mothers of infants with the fetal alcohol syndrome and found to be normal (4, 28). Possible effects of ethanol on intestinal absorption of folic acid have been reported by Halsted *et al.* (12). Hematologic response to folic acid therapy was prevented by the concomitant administration of whiskey, wine, or ethanol. Eichner and Hillman (7) found that when a folate-poor diet was given to alcoholics along with ethanol, megaloblastic changes developed much more rapidly than when the same diet was given to these subjects without alcohol. These findings suggest that alcohol administration causes megaloblastic changes only when body vitamin stores are decreased and dietary intake is poor. Under these circumstances, ethanol may act as a weak folate antagonist.

Studies on the effect on the rat embryo of maternal folate deficiency resulting from the administration of folate antagonists have shown that these agents may cause fetal resorption, stillbirths, and congenital malformations (13, 24, 25). In humans, a folic acid antagonist, aminopterin, can produce abortion (42). Recent reports suggest that human fetal malformations may also result from the administration of folate antagonists or from dietary deficiency of folate (10, 14). Therefore, the teratogenic effects of excessive alcohol ingestion during pregnancy may be due in some part to alcohol acting as a folic acid antagonist.

The work carried out by Victor *et al.* (46) at the Boston City Hospital showed that many of the central nervous system changes seen in adult alcoholics are probably due to thiamine deficiency. Consequently, thiamine deficiency in the mothers must be ruled out as a cause of the anomalies seen in the fetal alcohol syndrome. Neuropathologic changes in thiamine deficiency in adults have been found in the medial thalamic nuclei, mammillary bodies, periaqueductal gray matter and superior cerebellum (46). The clinical syndromes and localization of brain lesions seen in thiamine deficiency in postnatal life, however, bear no resemblance to abnormalities seen in the fetal alcohol syndrome.

Smoking

Although 20% of heavy drinking women in our study do not smoke, many are heavy smokers; however, we lack sufficient data to imply that heavy smoking is a possible contributing factor. Smoking has been associated with lowered infant birth weight (36). Rush and Kass (31) at the Boston City Hospital demonstrated a greater risk of prematurity and infant mortality in offspring of smoking mothers. To date, there is no evidence implicating smoking as a teratogenic influence.

Drug Abuse

Drug abuse was not prominent in any of the three drinking groups and was not reported by any of the mothers of infants with morphologic abnormalities. There are numerous reports of infants with congenital anomalies who were born to addict mothers, but there is no discernible pattern of anomalies in these infants and the incidence of congenital defects is not higher in offspring of addict mothers than in the general population (30).

Hypoglycemia

Hypoglycemia is known to follow ingestion of alcohol, and thus some of the abnormalities seen in the offspring of alcoholic women may be related to hypoglycemia early in the pregnancy. Infants of diabetic mothers have a much higher incidence of major congenital malformations than is seen in the general population, and hypoglycemia may play a significant role in the production of these abnormalities (11).

Deficiency of Trace Metals

Deficiency of trace metals is believed to play a role in the production of many illnesses affecting the nervous system. Magnesium and zinc deficiency are thought to have an effect in the production of Korsakoff syndrome with its attendant memory loss in the adult alcoholic (26, 41, 43). Whether these trace metals may be implicated in the production of the fetal alcohol syndrome is highly speculative in view of the fact that the fetus is often preferentially provided critical nutrients at the expense of the mother.

ANIMAL STUDIES OF EXPERIMENTAL ALCOHOLISM

Experimental work done on a number of pregnant animals given alcohol has resulted in low-birth-weight offspring with a significant number of central nervous system abnormalities.

Papara-Nicholson (29) fed ethanol to pregnant guinea pigs and produced offspring that were of low birth weight and had motor abnormalities, ataxia, and blindness. The brains of these animals showed flattened gyri, shallow sulci, and retarded myelinization. Sandor (32, 34) injected ethanol into chick embryos and noted a high incidence of malformations among the survivors, with defects of neural tube closure and rudimentary deformed brain vesicles. Ho *et al.* (15) gave radioactive labeled ethanol to pregnant hamsters and monkeys and demonstrated placental transfer of the ethanol with greater concentrations in later pregnancy. In the monkey, high concentrations were seen in the brain, especially in the visual cortex and cerebellum. The only report of experimental fetal alcoholism in the rat is by Sandor (33) who gave ethanol to rats early in pregnancy. Fetuses studied at 19½ days showed retarded skeletal development; there was, however, no description of the nervous system in these animals. Except for Sandor's findings of neural tube closure defects in chick embryos which suggests a teratogenic effect very early in the first trimester of pregnancy, both the clinical features in the human cases and the results of the experimental work in species other than the chick suggest a teratogenic effect somewhat later in the first trimester of pregnancy.

SUMMARY

The fetal alcohol syndrome has been described as microcephaly, micrognathia, microphthalamia, cardiac defects, and prenatal and postnatal growth retardation. In our study, prenatal growth retardation was present, but except for microcephaly in 2 patients, this consistent pattern of malformations was not found in the 15 offspring of heavy drinking mothers. All of the children described to date with the fetal alcohol syndrome have been born to severely alcoholic mothers, and most of these children have been identified only after a retrospective review. Although we identified 6 children in two families with multiple congenital anomalies consistent with the fetal alcohol syndrome and found an additional dozen unrelated cases by retrospective review, we have not demonstrated conclusively a specific pattern of anomalies among the offspring of heavy drinking women in our prospective study. Additional examinations on more infants will be necessary. It is likely that those infants heretofore identified represent the most severely afflicted infants at one end of a bell-shaped curve and that a spectrum of structural, growth, and functional abnormalities will be found in offspring of women with heavy alcohol intake during pregnancy. Because of the complexity of the interrelationships between excessive alcohol intake, smoking, drug abuse, poor nutrition, and other sociologic factors, large well-controlled prospective studies of this problem are essential if a true understanding is to be gained of the effects of maternal alcohol ingestion during pregnancy on the development of the child.

REFERENCES

1. Belfer ML, Shader RK, Carroll M, Harmatz JS: Alcoholism in women. Arch Gen Psychiatry 25:6, 540, 1971
2. Burton R: The Anatomy of Melancholy, Vol I. London, William Tegg, 1806, p 890
3. Cahalan D, Cisin IH, Crossley HM: American Drinking Practices: A National Study of Drinking Behavior and Attitudes. (Monograph No. 6). New Brunswick, NJ Rutgers Center of Alcohol Studies, 1969
4. Christiaens L, Miron LP, Delmarle G: Sur la descendance des alcooliques. Sem Hop Paris 36:257, 1960
5. Cravioto J, DeLicardie ER, Birch HC: Nutrition, growth and neurointegrative development: an experimental and ecologic study. Pediatrics 38(2):319, 1966
6. Criteria Committee, National Council on Alcoholism: Criteria for the diagnosis of alcoholism. Ann Intern Med 77:249, 1972
7. Eichner ER, Hillman RS: The evolution of anemia in alcoholic patients. Am J Med 50:218, 1971
8. Fielding H: An enquiry into the causes of the late increase of robbers, etc. with some proposal for remedying this growing evil. London, A Millar, 1751
9. Giroud A, Tuchmann–Duplessis H: Malformations congenitales, roles des facteurs exogenes. Pathol Biol 10:141, 1962
10. Goetsch C: An evaluation of aminopterin as an abortifacient. Am J Obstet Gynecol 83:1474, 1962
11. Gould J: Personal communication
12. Halsted CH, Griggs RC, Harris JW: The effect of alcoholism on the absorption of folic

acid (H³-PGA) evaluated by plasma levels and urine excretion. J Lab Clin Med 69:116, 1967

13. Hibbard BM: The role of folic acid in pregnancy, with particular reference to anaemia, abruption and abortion. J Obstet Gynaecol Br Commonw 71:529, 1964

14. Hibbard ED, Smithells RW: Folic acid metabolism and human embryopathy. Lancet 1:1254, 1965

15. Ho BT, Fritchie GE, Idanpaan–Heikkila JE, McIsaac WM: Placental transfer and tissue distribution of ethanol-1-¹⁴C. Q J Stud Alcohol 33:485, 1972

16. Jones KL, Smith DW: Recognition of the fetal alcohol syndrome in early infancy. Lancet 2:999, 1973

17. Jones KL, Smith DW, Streissguth AP, Myrianthopoulos NC: Incidence of the fetal alcohol syndrome in offspring of chronically alcoholic women. Pediatr Res 8:166, 1974

18. Jones KL, Smith DW, Streissguth AP, Myrianthopoulos NC: Outcome in offspring of chronic alcoholic women. Lancet 1:1076, 1974

19. Jones KL, Smith DW, Ulleland CN, Streissguth AP: Pattern of malformation in offspring of chronic alcoholic mothers. Lancet 1:1267, 1973

20. Lemoine P, Harousseau H, Borteyrn JP, Manure JC: Les enfants de parents alcooliques. Anomalies observees. Ouest–Medical 25:476, 1968

21. Miller JQ: Lissencephaly in 2 siblings. Neurology (Minneap) 13:841, 1963

22. Naeye RL, Blanc W, Paul C: Effects of maternal nutrition on the human fetus. Pediatrics 52:494, 1973

23. National Institute on Alcohol Abuse and Alcoholism. Washington DC, US Dept of Health, Education and Welfare, second report to US Congress, 1974

24. Nelson MM, Asling CW, Evans HM: Production of multiple congenital abnormalities in young by maternal pteroylglutamic acid deficiency during gestation. J Nutr 48:61, 1952

25. Nelson MM, Evans HM: Reproduction in rat on purified diets containing succinylsulfathiazole. Proc Soc Exp Biol Med 66:289, 1947

26. Oberleas D, Caldwell DF, Prasad AS: Trace elements and behavior. In Pfeiffer CC (ed): International Review of Neurobiology of Trace Metals Zinc and Copper. New York, Academic Press, 1972, pp 83–103

27. Ouellette EM: The fetal alcohol syndrome, additional familial cases. Madison, Proc 3rd Natl Meeting Child Neurol Soc, 1974

28. Palmer RH, Ouellette EM, Warner L, Leichtman SR: Congenital malformations in offspring of a chronic alcoholic mother. Pediatrics 53:490, 1974

29. Papara–Nicholson D, Telford IR: Effects of alcohol on reproduction and fetal development in the guinea pig. Anat Rec 127:438, 1957

30. Rothstein P, Gould JB: Born with a habit: infants of drug-addicted mothers. Pediatr Clin North Am 21:307, 1974

31. Rush D, Kass EH: Maternal smoking: a reassessment of the association with perinatal mortality. Am J Epidemiol 96:183, 1972

32. Sandor S: The influence of aethyl alcohol on the developing chick embryo. II. Rev Roum Embryol Cytol Ser Embryol 5:167, 1968

33. Sandor S, Amels D: The action of aethanol on the prenatal development of albino rats. (An attempt of multiphasic screening). Rev Roum Embryol Cytol Ser Embryol 8:105, 1971

34. Sandor S, Elias S: The influence of aethyl-alcohol on the development of the chick embryo. Rev Roum Embryol Cytol Ser Embryol 5:51, 1968

35. Sedgewick J: A new treatise on liquors, wherein the use and abuse of wine, malt-drinks, water, etc. are particularly consider'd in many diseases, constitutions and ages; with the proper manner of using them, hot, or cold, either as physick, diet or both. London, Charles Rivington, 1725

36. Simpson WJ: A preliminary report on cigarette smoking and the incidence of prematurity. Am J Obstet Gynecol 73:808, 1957

37. Smith CA: Effects of maternal undernutrition upon the newborn infant in Holland (1944–1945). J Pediatr 30:229, 1947
38. Stevens JP: Some of the effects of alcohol upon the physical constitution of man. South Med Surg J 13:451, 1857
39. Stoch MB, Smythe PM: Does undernutrition during infancy inhibit brain growth and subsequent intellectual development? Arch Dis Child 38:546, 1963
40. Stoch MB, Smythe PM: The effect of undernutrition during infancy on subsequent brain growth and intellectual development. South Afr Med J 41:1027, 1967
41. Sullivan JF, Lankford HG: Zinc metabolism in chronic alcoholism. Am J Clin Nutr 17:57, 1965
42. Thiersch JB: Therapeutic abortions with a folic acid antagonist, 4-aminopterolyl-glutamic acid (4-amino P.G.A.) administered by the oral route. Am J Obstet Gynecol 63:1298, 1952
43. Traviesa DC: Magnesium deficiency: a possible cause of thiamine refractoriness in Wernicke–Korsakoff encephalopathy. J Neurol Neurosurg Psychiatry 35:959, 1974
44. Triboulet H, Matthieu F, Mignot R: Traite de l'Alcoolisme. Paris, Masson et Cie, 1905
45. Ulleland CN: The offspring of alcoholic mothers. Ann NY Acad Sci 197:167, 1972
46. Victor M, Adams RD, Collins CH: The Wernicke–Korsakoff Syndrome. Philadelphia, FA Davis, 1971, p 147
47. Winick M: Malnutrition and brain development. J Pediatr 74:667, 1969
48. Winick M, Rosso P: Head circumference and cellular growth of the brain in normal and marasmic children. J Pediatr 74:774, 1969
49. Winick M, Rosso P: The effect of severe early malnutrition on cellular growth of human brain. Pediatr Res 3:181, 1969
50. Yakovlev PI: Morphological criteria of growth and maturation of the nervous system in man. Ment Retard 39:3, 1962

Chapter 10

Carbohydrate Metabolism—Some Aspects of Glycosuria

Tom Lind

In 1921 Bell (2), a surgeon from Detroit, suggested that, in pregnancy, glycosuria associated with a normal blood glucose level has a better prognosis than glycosuria with concomitant hyperglycemia. Two years later, Welz and Van Nest (21), also from Detroit, reported:

On the basis of numerous researches, it may now be said that the spontaneous and artificial glycosuria of pregnancy occurs without an important increase of blood sugar content. Hence this renal glycosuria of early pregnancy may be used to diagnose pregnancy during the first trimester.

These reports gave a strong indication that "benign" glycosuria was an interesting phenomenon which might be specific to pregnancy. Despite this, little attention has been paid to the nature and causes of glycosuria either during pregnancy or in diabetes. Indeed, it could be said that in pregnant women the exclusion of diabetes mellitus as a cause usually signals the end of interest in glycosuria.

The reasons why glucose may appear in urine during pregnancy are complex. Some of the changes in carbohydrate metabolism and renal function during pregnancy, with special reference to glycosuria, will be described in this chapter.

PREGNANCY AND PLASMA GLUCOSE HOMEOSTASIS

THE FASTING STATE

General

Most individuals, pregnant or nonpregnant, have a fairly stable fasting glucose level; but exactly how this concentration is determined and maintained is open to question. It is easy to postulate that the fall in blood glucose concentration from its peak value after a meal ceases to stimulate insulin secretion. At the pancreatic islet cells, a fall in insulin concentration probably allows an increased release of glucagon which, on reaching the liver, helps mobilize the conversion of glycogen to glucose. The role of glucagon in this respect has recently been emphasized (1). On the other hand, almost total suppression of insulin with infusions of growth-hormone release-inhibiting hormone (somatostatin) does not promote any significant rise in the fasting glucose level (17). There are other intriguing mysteries concerning the accurate "guarding" of the fasting glucose level. How is the control maintained? Why do some people have a fasting level of, say, 70 mg/100 ml and others 80 mg/100 ml? Why, if glucagon can mobilize blood glucose, does it stop at this individual, preset level in the fasting state? Most intriguing of all, however, why does the fasting blood glucose level, presumably the optimum for a given individual, change during pregnancy?

The Effect of Pregnancy

It is now widely accepted that the fasting plasma glucose concentration is lower during pregnancy (4, 13, 20). Lind *et al.* (13) did standard 50 g oral glucose tolerance tests (OGTTs) on 19 healthy women aged 20 to 32 years at 10, 20, 30, and 38 weeks of gestation and again at 10 to 12 weeks after delivery. This last test was taken as the nonpregnant response. The mean fasting values and standard deviations are given in Table 10–1; the fasting glucose concentration was significantly lower than the nonpregnant value at 10 weeks of gestation, but there was no significant downward trend thereafter. Thus, once homeostatic control is reset to the reduced level which characterizes pregnancy, it does not appear to alter. In an attempt to define more specifically when this change occurs, patients are being studied before conception, over the time of conception, and during the first 15 weeks of pregnancy. This work is still in progress, but it is possible to state that the reduced fasting blood glucose concentration is achieved gradually over the first 8 weeks or so of pregnancy and does not occur abruptly.

Fasting plasma insulin concentrations change in a different way during pregnancy (Table 10–1). The main feature is the rise towards the end of pregnancy, which, although small, is statistically significant. Because of these differences in timing, it is difficult to postulate a cause and effect relationship between lower fasting glucose levels and higher fasting insulin concentrations during pregnancy.

Virtually nothing is known about plasma glucagon changes during normal pregnancy. It is interesting to note that a recent book dealing exclusively with the molecular physiology of glucagon and its clinical and therapeutic implications does not mention pregnancy at all (12). While the resetting of the fasting glucose concentration in an individual may well represent a new balance between insulin and glucagon at the liver cell, this is only conjecture at the present time.

Table 10–1. MEAN FASTING PLASMA GLUCOSE AND INSULIN CONCENTRATIONS (±SD) IN 19 WOMEN THROUGHOUT PREGNANCY AND ABOUT 10 WEEKS AFTER DELIVERY*

Fasting plasma sample	PD	Weeks of pregnancy			
		10	20	30	38
Glucose	79.8	75.0	71.1	74.3	68.8
(mg/100 ml)	±5.7	±8.3	±7.2	±7.2	±7.7
Insulin	5.8	4.2	4.2	7.6	7.8
(μU/ml)	±4.0	±2.4	±1.8	±2.9	±3.8

PD, test performed about 10 weeks after delivery and representing the nonpregnant level.
*Lind T, Billewicz WZ, Brown G: J Obstet Gynaecol Br Commonw 80:1033, 1973

THE FED STATE

General

The most commonly used test for determining the response of an individual to a carbohydrate load is the 50 g oral glucose tolerance test. Under normal circumstances, few people break a fast by drinking 50 g of glucose and in this respect the test could be regarded as unphysiologic, but for the purposes of discussion only, OGTT data will be considered. It is still the least artificial of the standard tests for the investigation of carbohydrate metabolism.

After drinking a glucose load the blood glucose will increase during the first hour and by 2–2½ hours will have returned to the fasting level again. Some books indicate that the peak value might occur before 1 hour, and that at 2 hours or more the concentration might fall slightly below the pretest fasting level (18). Our experience has been that the response to an oral load of glucose shows a wide spectrum of behavior and varies considerably between individuals. Smoothed mean plasma glucose and insulin response curves of the 19 women previously described are shown in Figure 10–1. The samples were taken at 15-minute intervals for 90 minutes and, therefore, allow more precise individual response curves to be drawn. In young, healthy nonpregnant women, the peak glucose value occurs about 30 minutes after drinking the glucose, and the fasting value is regained at about 60 minutes. In some subjects, the plasma glucose concentration fell appreciably below the fasting value before 2 hours.

Some women show only a trivial rise in the plasma glucose concentration following the glucose drink. However, such patients have an insulin response

Fig. 10–1. The mean glucose and insulin response curves during oral glucose tolerance tests performed at 38 weeks' gestation and after delivery (labelled non-pregnant). (Lind T, Billewicz WZ, Brown G: J Obstet Gynaecol Br Commonw 80:1033, 1973)

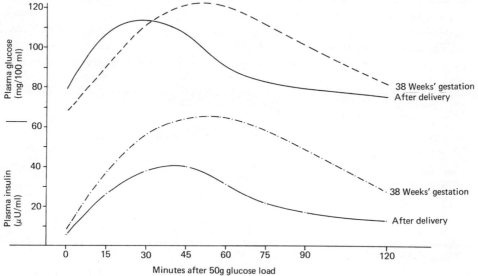

which is as brisk as in those with a more "normal" glucose response. It may be that absorption occurs normally, but the rate of diffusion from the plasma into the total extracellular space and tissue uptake is so rapid that the effective "plasma pool" hardly increases above the fasting state.

Another type of response is characterized by a secondary rise in plasma glucose concentration after the initial peak has been passed. This is usually much less than the peak value but too high to be accounted for by laboratory variation in glucose determination. That this secondary rise is genuine is confirmed by a corresponding insulin response. Because of such variations, diagnoses based on blood glucose values at set time points, such as the concentrations at 2 hours as advocated in the WHO (1965) definition of diabetes (22), may be misleading.

The insulin response reaches its maximum value slightly after the glucose peak, but the shape of the response curve is similar, and again the fasting value is usually achieved at or before 2 hours. The fasting value for healthy individuals is about 6 μU/ml. With a sensitive immunoassay, values as low as 2 μU/ml can be confidently determined, and from our data, it seems that the insulin concentration does not fall much below the fasting value in the course of an OGTT.

The Effect of Pregnancy

As pregnancy progresses, the time to reach the maximum glucose concentration becomes longer. By 38 weeks of gestation in the subjects studied (13), the mean time to the peak plasma glucose level was 55 minutes as compared to the nonpregnant value of 34 minutes. Despite this, the fasting level was still achieved in most cases by 2 hours. The actual concentration achieved was also somewhat higher than in the nonpregnant state; taken in conjunction with the lower starting, or fasting, value, this means that pregnant women have a higher incremental plasma glucose. These changes can be quantified in two ways: the total or incremental areas under the response curve can be determined in arbitrary units (10); or the *shape* of the curve can be expressed as a number using the *H index* (3).

The effect of pregnancy on the insulin response is even more striking. The peak value becomes progressively higher, and the time to reach this value is

Table 10–2. ESTIMATED TIME TO REACH MAXIMUM GLUCOSE AND INSULIN CONCENTRATIONS IN THE COURSE OF A 50-g ORAL GLUCOSE TOLERANCE TEST AT VARIOUS STAGES OF PREGNANCY*

Stage of Pregnancy	Mean peak time ±SD (mins)	
	Glucose	Insulin
Gestation (wks)		
10	33.9 ± 15.2	39.7 ± 13.7
20	36.9 ± 15.2	45.6 ± 13.6
30	44.1 ± 16.3	51.1 ± 17.5
38	54.9 ± 15.3	58.2 ± 15.7
Postdelivery	32.5 ± 13.6	41.7 ± 11.1

*Lind T, Billewicz WZ, Brown G: J Obstet Gynaecol Br Commonw 80:1033, 1973

Table 10–3. MEAN GLUCOSE AND INSULIN CONCENTRATION DURING THE COURSE OF ORAL GLUCOSE TOLERANCE TESTS IN 19 HEALTHY WOMEN THROUGHOUT PREGNANCY AND AT 10 WEEKS POSTDELIVERY*

Sampling time (min)	Gestation (wks)									
	Glucose (mg/100 ml)					Insulin (μU/ml)				
	PD	10	20	30	38	PD	10	20	30	38
0	79.8 ± 5.7	75.0 ± 8.3	71.1 ± 7.2	74.3 ± 7.2	68.8 ± 7.7	5.8 ± 4.0	4.2 ± 2.4	4.2 ± 1.8	7.6 ± 2.9	7.8 ± 3.8
15	109.8 ±11.7	104.9 ±14.9	95.4 ±11.4	101.3 ±16.0	89.7 ±12.8	27.7 ±18.2	28.3 ±24.8	27.6 ±13.9	37.1 ±21.7	37.7 ±29.3
30	114.8 ±19.3	112.3 ±21.5	105.5 ±18.9	119.1 ±23.4	113.1 ±15.5	38.8 ±18.0	41.4 ±24.9	40.4 ±25.2	55.9 ±37.9	57.6 ±35.7
45	109.0 ±22.5	111.9 ±24.0	107.1 ±23.8	122.3 ±28.8	121.7 ±20.7	42.0 ±18.8	42.6 ±25.0	45.3 ±21.7	67.1 ±39.7	63.0 ±26.0
60	91.1 ±21.4	100.2 ±26.7	99.2 ±23.0	111.7 ±24.2	121.5 ±19.7	32.7 ±16.1	34.8 ±19.7	38.7 ±18.8	61.4 ±36.8	66.4 ±35.2
75	85.1 ±20.5	93.9 ±18.9	93.0 ±20.7	101.2 ±22.8	111.3 ±20.9	23.2 ±12.8	31.4 ±20.3	34.3 ±15.0	52.8 ±32.4	56.8 ±22.8
90	82.5 ±16.7	89.4 ±22.6	83.5 ±23.6	96.6 ±22.2	102.5 ±19.9	19.5 ±10.8	32.0 ±40.2	23.4 ±14.3	40.6 ±19.6	51.6 ±24.2
120	77.4 ±19.7	87.1 ±23.0	70.8 ±17.5	79.1 ±17.0	81.3 ±18.3	13.4 ±12.5	16.9 ±12.6	15.8 ±11.0	22.7 ±17.2	28.2 ±14.9

PD, tests performed 10 weeks after delivery.
*Lind T, Billewicz WZ, Brown G: J Obstet Gynaecol Br Commonw 80:1033, 1973

delayed. By 2 hours the insulin concentration is usually still well above the fasting concentration (Fig. 10–1; Table 10–2). The plasma glucose and insulin data for each test and all time intervals obtained from the 19 women followed regularly throughout pregnancy are given in Table 10–3.

It is thus obvious that normal pregnancy in healthy women considerably modifies glucose and insulin homeostasis and that the effect is progressive as pregnancy advances. To ensure that our postnatal test is indicative of the non-pregnant state, the OGTT is repeated at a minimum of 6 weeks and usually 8–10 weeks postpartum, but it is probable that the effect of pregnancy on glucose homeostasis has disappeared much earlier than this. Indeed, Lund and Weese (16) commented that one of the difficulties of detecting gestational diabetes retrospectively is that the curve often reverts to normal within 48 hours of delivery.

It could be argued that the insulin response in each pregnant individual is the maximum of which she is capable but that this maximum response is inadequate during pregnancy; hence the "diabetogenic" effect in some pregnancies. This explanation is untenable. During the course of experiments performed to determine the glomerular filtration rate (GFR) during pregnancy, 10 healthy normal pregnant women were infused with 10% dextrose solution. The mean plasma glucose and insulin concentrations achieved at each stage of pregnancy are given in Table 10–4. As shown, these women were capable of a massive insulin response under infusion conditions.

MATERNAL AND CORD BLOOD GLUCOSE AND INSULIN RELATIONS

Glucose and insulin levels in 854 cord blood samples and 503 concurrently collected maternal blood samples were measured (14); 236 of the mothers had received a sugar-containing fluid during labor, usually as a carrier for oxytocin.

Table 10–4. PLASMA GLUCOSE AND INSULIN CONCENTRATIONS DURING GLUCOSE INFUSIONS THROUGHOUT PREGNANCY IN 10 PATIENTS

| Gestatation | Duration of infusion (mins) | | | |
	0	40	60	80
PD				
PG	88	229	221	229
PI	5.7	35.1	48.9	66.4
16 Wks				
PG	75	179	175	174
PI	6.6	79.5	87.5	89.5
26 Wks				
PG	78	194	192	195
PI	12.7	93.0	94.2	115.6
36 Wks				
PG	82	199	210	213
PI	16.0	130.2	163.2	198.6

PG, plasma glucose (mg/100 ml), PI, plasma insulin (μU/ml), PD, after delivery.

Excluding all cases of diabetes, the mean cord insulin level was 7 μU/ml—or 8 μU/ml if the mother received intravenous fluids. The distribution was markedly skewed with concentrations of 30 μU/ml or more in 12 infants (Fig. 10–2). Variables such as intravenous fluids during labor, birth weight, and type of delivery did not account for the wide range of cord insulin values.

While maternal hyperglycemia might be the most important cause of hyperinsulinism in neonates born to diabetic mothers, it seems not to be so in normal (nondiabetic) cases, there being virtually no relation between maternal or cord glucose values and cord insulin concentrations. It seems reasonable to infer that, in normal cases, some other factor is stimulating some fetuses to produce much more insulin than others.

PREGNANCY AND GLUCOSE EXCRETION

Glucose is filtered from the plasma in the glomerulus and reabsorbed in the proximal tubule. "Glycosuria" can result from an increase in plasma glucose concentration, an increase in the volume of blood filtered per minute, a decrease in the amount absorbed, or some combination of these factors. Clinicians usually interpret glycosuria as indicating hyperglycemia, though the use of the term *lowered renal threshold* implies that pregnancy can be associated with glycosuria in the presence of a "normal" plasma glucose level. We began to study glycosuria in an attempt to explain its characteristics and causes in healthy pregnant women. A brief description of renal adaptations during pregnancy might be helpful.

Fig. 10–2. Percentage distribution of cord plasma insulin values (854 cases). (Lind T, Gilmore EA, McClarence M: Br J Obstet Gynaecol 82:562, 1975)

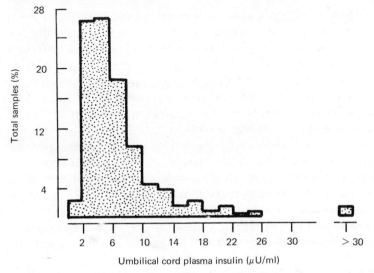

GLOMERULAR FILTRATION RATE

The glomerular filtration rate increases rapidly during the first 8 weeks of pregnancy to about 50% above the normal nonpregnant level (5). Thus, if the plasma glucose concentration remains constant, an increase of the GFR by itself will mean the presentation to the renal tubules of 50% more glucose which must be resorbed if detectable glycosuria is not to occur. But we have already noted that the postprandial rise of blood glucose is elevated and prolonged during pregnancy, and this further increases the filtered load presented to the tubules.

TUBULAR REABSORPTION

The traditional idea that in the healthy person all filtered glucose is resorbed is no longer tenable. The development of highly accurate and specific enzymatic methods for determining glucose in urine has shown that we all excrete some glucose in urine though this is usually less than 100 mg/24 hours (15). Under infusion conditions it can be shown that with increasing plasma glucose concentrations, and hence increased filtered loads, the tubules absorb more and more glucose but with decreasing efficiency. Thus plotting the filtered glucose load against the amount resorbed produces a curve (7) and not the classic plateau (often called the Tm_G threshold). It now seems very doubtful that the concept of a Tm_G, the maximum tubular resorptive capacity for glucose, which is constant and characteristic in any individual (19), has any basis in reality (16).

Everything said so far would apply equally well to substances other than glucose which are filtered by the glomerulus and have to be resorbed, for example, amino acids (9) and folate (11).

GLYCOSURIA OF NORMAL PREGNANCY

In an attempt to define the amount and pattern of glucose excretion during pregnancy, 30 healthy pregnant women were asked to test each sample of urine they passed for 1 week/month and on the seventh day of each week to collect all the urine over an exact 24 hours so that the total excretion could be determined (15). It was found that 10 women had no increase in their glucose excretion through pregnancy above the "normal" nonpregnant value of 100 mg/24 hours; the remainder excreted more than 100 mg/24 hours on some days, and 10 women excreted more than 1000 mg on at least 1 day.

The variables encountered, both per 24 hours and within single days, are illustrated in Figures 10–3 and 10–4 which show results from 2 patients.

Glycosuria occurred more frequently after meals, particularly in the evening, but there were so many exceptions that no convincing relationship could be postulated. Each patient had a normal OGTT.

In a further study, we found that, irrespective of the degree of glycosuria, all patients had returned to a normal glucose excretion level by the sixth day of the puerperium (8).

Such findings cannot be explained without revising the classic views on how

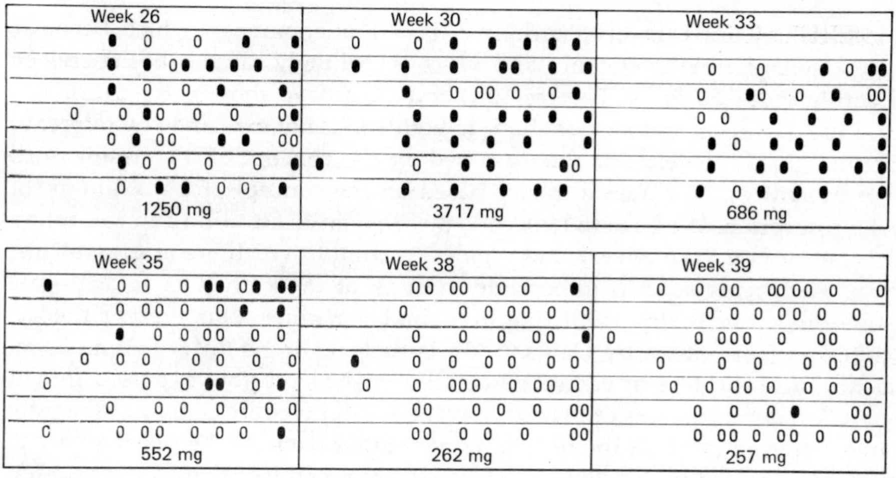

Fig. 10–3. Pattern of glycosuria in late pregnancy, as evidenced by Clinistix testing in 1 subject. The six blocks each represent 1 week of gestation (actual week specified above each block) divided horizontally into 7 days, midnight to midnight. Each sample of urine passed is indicated by a circle placed at the appropriate time on the scale. Solid circles are those which were positive to Clinistix. On the seventh day of each week the urine was collected and the total glucose excreted was estimated, the figure in milligrams is that total. (Lind T, Hytten FE: J Obstet Gynaecol Br Commonw 79:961, 1972)

Fig. 10–4. Pattern of glycosuria in late pregnancy, as evidenced by Clinistix testing in a further subject (details as in Fig. 3). (Lind T, Hytten FE: J Obstet Gynaecol Br Commonw 79: 961, 1972)

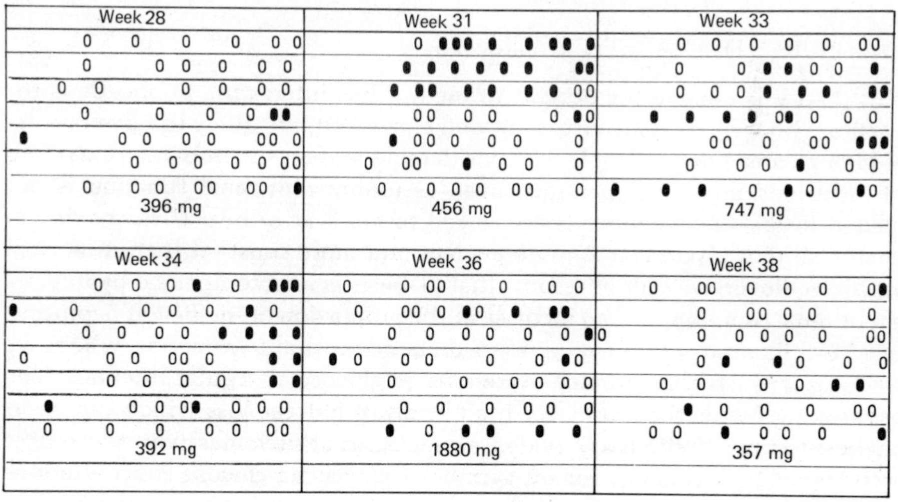

the kidney functions. In glycosuria, we have a phenomenon which becomes exaggerated by normal pregnancy and which is strikingly variable both between and within individuals. As Figures 10–3 and 10–4 have shown, glycosuria can appear and disappear almost from hour to hour and is not explained by reference to plasma glucose levels. No theory based on the concept of a constant renal threshold suffices. Nor does a theory based on the concept of a maximum for tubular resorption. We have to look for a mechanism of filtration and resorption which can respond sensitively and rapidly to stimuli which are at present unknown. That being so, it is impossible to think of the kidney as an aggregate of nephrons all of which are acting in a similar manner. Our present theory, described in more detail by Davison (6), is that nephrons differ in functional efficiency, and short-term variations of intrarenal blood flow expose different glomeruli to differing rates of plasma flow; hence, tubules are exposed to rapidly varying filtration rates. In the normal nonpregnant woman, the plasma flow to each glomerulus, and the proportion filtered, are much less than the maximum possible, and in general all nephrons are "ticking over" at a capacity well below the capacity of the most efficient and within the capability of even the least efficient. Pregnancy, by raising plasma flow and glomerular filtration rates, together with its effect on blood glucose homeostasis, completely alters the picture. Nephrons with a large reabsorptive capacity will still be capable of dealing with the increased filtered load, but other nephrons will fail to reabsorb glucose completely so that glycosuria appears. However, changes of blood flow within the kidney still occur and account for the variability of glycosuria as it appears clinically. Glucose infusion may cause maximal perfusion of all nephrons with consequent full exposure of the inadequacies of the less efficient tubules.

GLYCOSURIA IN DIABETIC PATIENTS

If this theory is tenable for normal women, it has interesting implications for diabetics who, even if their disease is well controlled, are likely to have unusually high plasma glucose levels for considerable lengths of time in any day. As with infusions in normal patients, even assuming that renal function is not impaired in diabetics, nephrons are forced to work at or near their maximum capacity, so that glycosuria is more evident and more constant than in normal women. However, we cannot assume that diabetes is unaccompanied by impairment of renal function, e.g., an increase in the proportion of inefficient nephrons. Table 10–5 illustrates two examples of diabetic pregnant women in whom we have measured 24-hour urinary excretions of glucose at regular intervals. The most striking fact is the extremely high levels of glucose loss which can occur from time to time. Preliminary evidence suggests that such massive and variable losses cannot be accounted for by variations in plasma glucose concentrations or GFR. It seems probable that diabetes is accompanied by functional impairment in a heterogenous assemblage of nephrons.

Table 10–5. 24-HOUR EXCRETION OF GLUCOSE IN 2 PREGNANT DIA-
BETIC PATIENTS DETERMINED AT REGULAR INTERVALS
BETWEEN 35 AND 37 WEEKS OF GESTATION

Urine volume (ml/24 hrs)		Urine glucose (g/24 hrs)	
Mrs. M	Mrs. H	Mrs. M	Mrs. H
1500	2100	44.8	11.8
2000	1500	21.0	2.7
1450	2750	33.0	100.1
1500	1400	31.2	0.4
950	2500	1.6	38.7

Average interval between samples was 4 days.

NUTRITIONAL CONSIDERATIONS

About half of all normal healthy women excrete above average amounts of glucose in their urine during normal pregnancy. As it seems unlikely that such losses can be explained by renal mechanisms which affect glucose only, it seems reasonable to conclude that such women also excrete increased amounts of water-soluble vitamins and amino acids. We know that excretion of such substances does increase during pregnancy (9, 11), but we do not know whether it is associated with increased glucose losses.

In women from a well-fed community with good social standards, it seems unlikely that renal losses of nutrients would lead to any significant impairment of maternal health or fetal well-being. On the other hand, in women from chronically malnourished populations, such physiologic losses might be sufficient to impair their already insufficient nutrient status to a degree where the fetus is put at hazard. In such a situation the detection of persistent glycosuria may be an indication for nutritional supplementation as well as for the investigation of possible diabetes mellitus.

The proven diabetic patient poses a special problem. The presence of glycosuria in such patients has for long been recognized as a part of their clinical picture, but it has perhaps not been sufficiently considered as a possible cause of undernutrition and malnutrition where renal losses of nutrients are large. It seems that losses of 20–30 g/24 hours can occur but are probably tolerable in an otherwise "stable" patient. From time to time, however, losses may be so great as to necessitate dietary supplementation. If the urinary losses of other essential nutrients in pregnant diabetics are proportionally as great as those of glucose, the total effect upon the mother and fetus *in utero* may well be sufficient to impair the obstetric outcome still further.

REFERENCES

1. Alford FP, Bloom SR, Nabarro JDN, Hall R, Besser GM, Coy DH, Kastin AJ, Schally AV: Glucagon control of fasting glucose in man. Lancet 2:974, 1974
2. Bell JN: Diabetes and pregnancy. Am J Obstet Gynecol 3:20, 1922
3. Billewicz WZ, Anderson J, Lind T: New index for evaluation of oral glucose tolerance test results. Br Med J 1:573, 1973
4. Bleicher SJ, O'Sullivan JB, Freinkel N: Carbohydrate metabolism in pregnancy. V. The interrelations of glucose, insulin and free fatty acids in late pregnancy and post-partum. N Engl J Med 271:866, 1964
5. Davison JM: Changes in renal function and other aspects of homeostasis in early pregnancy. J Obstet Gynaecol Br Commonw 81:1003, 1974
6. Davison JM: Renal nutrient excretion with emphasis on glucose. In Hytten FE (ed): Clinics in Obstetrics and Gynaecology. Vol 2. Physiological Adjustments in Pregnancy. Philadelphia, WB Saunders, 1975, pp 365–380
7. Davison JM, Hytten FE: Renal handling of glucose. In Sutherland HW, Stowers JM (eds): Carbohydrate Metabolism in Pregnancy and the Newborn. New York, Churchill Livingstone, 1975, pp 2–18
8. Davison JM, Lovedale C: The excretion of glucose during normal pregnancy and after delivery. J Obstet Gynaecol Br Commonw 81:30, 1974
9. Hytten FE, Cheyne GA: The aminoaciduria of pregnancy. J Obstet Gynaecol Br Commonw 79:424, 1972
10. Jarrett RJ, Graver HJ: Changes in oral glucose tolerance during the menstrual cycle. Br Med J 2:528, 1968
11. Landon MJ: Folate metabolism in pregnancy. In Hytten FE (ed): Clinics in Obstetrics and Gynaecology. Vol 2. Physiological Adjustments in Pregnancy. Philadelphia, WB Saunders, 1975, pp 413–430
12. Lefebure PJ, Unger RH: Glucagon, Molecular Physiology, Clinical and Therapeutic Implications. Oxford, Pergamon, 1972
13. Lind T, Billewicz WZ, Brown G: A serial study of changes occurring in the oral glucose tolerance test during pregnancy. J Obstet Gynaecol Br Commonw 80:1033, 1973
14. Lind T, Gilmore EA, McClarence M: Cord plasma glucose and insulin concentrations and maternal-fetal relations. Br J Obstet Gynaecol 82:562, 1975
15. Lind T, Hytten FE: The excretion of glucose during normal pregnancy. J Obstet Gynaecol Br Commonw 79:961, 1972
16. Lund CJ, Weese WH: Glucose tolerance and excessively large babies in nondiabetic mothers. Am J Obstet Gynecol 65:815, 1953
17. Mortimer CH, Carr D, Lind T, Bloom SR, Mallinson CN, Schally AV, Tunbridge WMG, Yeomans L, Coy DH, Kastin A, Besser GM, Hall R: Effects of growth-hormone release-inhibiting hormone on circulating glucagon, insulin and growth hormone in normal, diabetic, acromegalic and hypopituitary patients. Lancet 1:697, 1974
18. Passmore R, Robson JS: A Companion to Medical Studies, Vol 1. Oxford, Blackwell Scientific, 1968
19. Smith HW, Goldring W, Chasis H, Ranges HA, Bradley SE: The application of saturation methods to the study of glomerular and tubular function in the human kidney. Mt Sinai J Med NY 10:59, 1943
20. Tyson JE, Merimee TJ: Some physiologic effects of protein ingestion in pregnancy. Am J Obstet Gynecol 107:797, 1970
21. Welz WE, Van Nest AE: Sugar test in pregnancy. Am J Obstet Gynecol 5:33, 1923
22. WHO Expert Committee: Diabetes Mellitus. (Tech Rep No. 310:5). Geneva, 1965

Chapter 11

Maternal Nutrition—Its Effects on Infant Growth and Development and Birthspacing

Hernan Delgado, Aaron Lechtig, Charles Yarbrough, Reynaldo Martorell, Robert E. Klein, Marc Irwin

The prevalence of low-birth-weight infants ($\leqslant 2.5$ kg) ranges between 13% and 43% in the low socioeconomic groups of many countries (38). Moreover, the frequency of physical growth retardation during the first year of life is widespread. These babies have a low survival rate during the first year of life and perform poorly on mental development tests (8, 9). It is widely believed that environmental factors account for most growth failures, developmental retardation, and high mortality rates.

Maternal and child malnutrition has been implicated as one of several environmental factors capable of producing these high rates of growth, developmental retardation and infant mortality. Moreover, several investigators have postulated that environmental factors such as health and nutritional status affect the duration of birth interval (25, 27, 55). However, this assertion is difficult to substantiate because of the imprecision involved in defining maternal and child nutritional status and because of a lack of information concerning the effects of several factors which may constitute alternative explanations of the detected associations.

This chapter examines alternative explanations through a food supplementation study which was carried out in a chronically malnourished population. The effect of food supplementation during pregnancy and lactation on 1) fetal growth, 2) infant growth, 3) psychologic test performance, and 4) infant mortality in the study population will be reported in addition to environmental factors correlated with the duration of birth interval.

INSTITUTE OF NUTRITION OF CENTRAL AMERICA AND PANAMA LONGITUDINAL STUDY

The Institute's longitudinal study has been well described elsewhere (16, 33); however, a brief description follows.

*This research was supported by Contract N01-HD-5-0640 from the National Institute of Child Health and Human Development, National Institutes of Health, Bethesda, Md.

POPULATION

In 1969, a longitudinal study of the biologic and socioeconomic determinants of physical growth and mental development in rural Guatemala was begun. The project involved four small villages of eastern Guatemala. The ethnic background of the population is Ladino, or mixed Indian and Spanish. These are agricultural villages, and the main crops are corn and beans, most of which are consumed in the same village. Houses are built from material obtained locally, mainly adobe, and consist of two rooms, one of which is used as sleeping quarters by the whole family. The total population of the four villages is about 3500, half of the inhabitants being below 15 years of age. The number of previous deliveries among the women studied range between 0 and 12, and the reproductive span is from age 14 to 46. Approximately 160 children are born each year in the four villages combined.

There is little permanent migration, and contact with the outside world is limited to trips to nearby markets. Seasonal migration occurs once a year when some of the men harvest cash crops in the coastal zone. The median annual income is approximately $200.00 per family, with most expenditures allocated for food and clothing. Modern contraceptive practices are uncommon. Sanitary conditions are poor, leading to a high prevalence of infectious diseases, especially those of diarrheal nature. Drinking water is obtained from wells or a creek, and only 6% of the houses have latrines. Within the study villages, moderate malnutrition is endemic.

DESIGN

The basic hypothesis of this study was that mild to moderate protein-calorie malnutrition adversely affects the mental development of infants and preschool-aged children. To test the hypothesis, a quasi-experimental design was employed. Experimental treatment consisted of food supplementation in four closely matched villages. In two of the villages, a high protein-calorie supplementation drink was made available daily in a central dispensary. This beverage is similar to a popular local gruel, *atole*. In the other two villages, a non-protein, low-calorie drink similar to a local cold drink known as *fresco* was provided daily. The nutrient content of both supplements is shown in Table 11–1.

The low-calorie beverage, or fresco, contained no protein and provided only one-third of the calories contained in an equal volume of atole. Both supplements contained the vitamins, minerals, and fluoride which were limited in the normal diet. The subjects under study were children 7 years old and under, and all pregnant and lactating women in the four villages. Since consumption of the supplements was voluntary, a wide range of supplement intake during pregnancy and lactation in mothers and in infants was observed. In addition to dietary supplementation, all four villages received preventive and curative medical care.

Table 11–1. NUTRIENT CONTENT PER CUP* (180 ML) OF SUPPLEMENTATION DRINK

	Atole†	Fresco‡
Total calories (kcal)	163	59
Protein (g)	11	—
Fats (g)	0.7	—
Carbohydrates (g)	27	15.3
Ascorbic acid (mg)	4.0	4.0
Calcium (g)	0.4	—
Phosphorus (g)	0.3	—
Thiamine (mg)	1.1	1.1
Riboflavin (mg)	1.5	1.5
Niacin (mg)	18.5	18.5
Vitamin A (mg)	1.2	1.2
Iron (mg)	5.4	5.0
Fluor (mg)	0.2	0.2

*Review date: October 11, 1973; figures rounded to the nearest tenth.
†The name of a gruel commonly made with corn.
‡Spanish for refreshing, cool drink.

Table 11–2. DATA COLLECTED IN INCAP LONGITUDINAL STUDY

Maternal and child information

Independent variable:

    Measurements of subject's attendance to feeding
    center and amount of supplement ingested

Dependent variables:

    Assessment of physical growth
    Assessment of mental development
    Infant mortality
    Birth Interval

Additional variables:

    Obstetric history*
    Information on delivery
    Clinical examination
    Dietary survey
    Morbidity survey
    Socioeconomic survey of the family

*Diagnosis of pregnancy by absence of menstruation.

METHODS

The principal examinations made during the prenatal and postnatal period are presented in Table 11–2. Data collected were standardized carefully, and the data collectors were systematically rotated among the four study villages.

Ingestion of additional calories was selected as the criteria to assess supplement intake because the home diet appeared to be more limited in calories than in proteins. The variables were the prevalence of physical growth retardation at birth and 6 months of age, psychologic test performance at birth and 6 months of age, infant mortality, and birth interval.

In the study population, the protein/calorie ratio in the home diet is approximately 11%. Thus, we believe it is feasible to improve the total diet of mothers by adding more calories. While calories appear to be limited in this study population, other populations may present very different nutritional situations.

In the following analyses, caloric intake since conception will be expressed as both a continuous and a discrete variable. Two continuous variables are employed, maternal caloric intake during pregnancy and intake during lactation. In some analyses, these two components are combined into one summary variable. The limits defining the categories comprising the discrete variables are presented in Table 11–3.

Up to 6 months of age, the categorization of nutritional status depends only on the intake of the mother. Except for the rare case of severe maternal illness, all children are breast-fed to the age of 6 months and most do not receive supplementary foods. In constructing long-term categories, it was found that the sample sizes for the high-calorie supplement group would be very small if it were required that the mother be in the group during all three trimesters. Consequently, high-calorie supplemented children were defined as those well-supplemented during 75% of the periods. This definition is considered sufficiently strict to generate useful nutritional status evaluations.

Table 11–4 presents the sample sizes for each of the variables examined. The total sample included 671 births which occurred in the four villages from January 1969 through February 1973.

EFFECT OF MATERNAL NUTRITION ON FETAL GROWTH

The effect of maternal nutrition on birth weight under situations of acute starvation is clearly established (1, 28, 54). On the other hand, studies concerning the influence of chronic moderate malnutrition on fetal growth have shown less

Table 11–3. DEFINITION OF LOW, INTERMEDIATE AND HIGH CALORIC SUPPLEMENTATION STATUS SINCE CONCEPTION

1. Description of the Scoring for Each Time Interval

Time intervals (months)	Subject	Criteria to be defined as: (Supplemented Calories in thousands)		
		Low	Intermediate	High
Pregnancy	Mother	< 10	10–19.9	≥ 20
0–3	Mother	< 5	5– 9.9	≥ 10
3–6	Mother	< 5	5– 9.9	≥ 10

2. Summary Periods	**Total Number of Time Intervals**	**Minimum No. of Time Intervals in the same category**
1. Pregnancy	2	2 (100%)
2. Conception to 6 months	4	3 (75%)

3. An infant is classified as Low or High if his mother has ranked in the same category for at least 75% of the time intervals. If not, he is classified as Intermediate.

Table 11–4. SAMPLE SIZE FOR VARIABLES EXAMINED

Variable	Number of children born into sample
Children Available*	671
Physical growth	
At birth	405
At 6 months	447
Mental development	
At birth	157
At 6 months	472
Infant mortality (first 12 months of age)	653†
Birth interval (post-partum amenorrhea and lactation; entirely prospective and followed during entire interval)	334‡

*Births which occurred in the four villages from January 1, 1969 through February 28, 1973.
†Up to February 28, 1974.
‡Up to November 30, 1974.

Table 11–5. BIRTH WEIGHT BY THREE CATEGORIES OF MATERNAL CALORIC SUPPLEMENTATION DURING PREGNANCY

| | Level of maternal caloric supplementation | | | |
	Low	Intermediate	High	t test (high–low)
Mean birth weight (g)	2986	3036	3120	2.62*
Percent low birthweight (≤ 2.5 kg)	18.30	15.85	9.41	2.33†
Number of infants	153	82	170	

*$P \leq 0.01$.
†$P \leq 0.05$; t test, after arc sine transformation of percentage values.

Table 11–6. RELATIONSHIP BETWEEN DIFFERENCES IN CALORIC SUPPLEMENTATION DURING PREGNANCY AND DIFFERENCES IN BIRTH WEIGHT FOR TWO CONSECUTIVE SIBLINGS (LATTER MINUS PRECEDING PREGNANCY)

Differences in caloric supplementation categories	Difference in birth weights (mean ± SD) (g)	No. of sibling pairs
−40,000 − 0 cal	−172 ± 586	25
100 − 20,000 cal	20 ± 469	35
20,100 − 120,000 cal	218 ± 355	34

t Test (high–low) = 2.95; P < .01.

clear results. Although it has been demonstrated that maternal size before pregnancy and weight gain during pregnancy show consistent associations with
birth weight, and that these relationships may reflect the influence of the maternal nutrition status on fetal growth (49), several studies using information from
dietary surveys or food supplementation programs have failed to find an association between nutrient intake during pregnancy and birth weight (20, 48, 56).
On the other hand, in studies showing an association between maternal nutritional intake and birth weight (7, 22, 41, 46), the influence of potentially confounding variables such as size of the mother, presence of infectious disease, and
physical activity has not been explicitly controlled.

In the INCAP study, we found a consistently high association between maternal nutrition during pregnancy and birth weight (37, 38, 42, 43).

Table 11–5 shows the mean birth weight and percentage of low-birth-weight
babies ($\leqslant$ 2.5 kg) by three categories of maternal supplement ingestion. The
low-calorie group consists of mothers whose total ingestion during pregnancy
was less than 10,000 calories, while the high-calorie group consists of mothers
whose ingestion was greater than or equal to 20,000 calories. The proportion of
low-birth-weight babies was consistently lower in the better supplemented
group in both fresco- and atole-consuming populations. Thus, the risk of deliv-
ering low-birth-weight babies among high supplemented mothers was roughly
half that of the low supplemented group. However, since home caloric intake
was similar in both groups, we have concluded that the supplemental calories
were additional to the basic maternal diet. In the high-calorie supplementation
group, this addition amounted to about 35,000 calories during all of pregnancy,
or about 125 cal/day extra.

The possibility that confounding factors could be responsible for the association observed between caloric supplementation and birth weight was studied.
Findings indicate that this association is not explained by other maternal variables related to birth weight such as size, home diet, morbidity, obstetrical characteristics, and socioeconomic status. Furthermore, the association between caloric supplementation and birth weight was not produced by undetected
confounding factors related to the mother (*i.e.*, a tendency to have bigger babies), since it was also observed within two consecutive siblings of the same
mother.

Table 11–6 points out the differences in birth weight for 94 pairs of siblings
divided into three supplementation groups.

These groups were defined by differences in caloric supplementation of the
mother between two successive pregnancies. When caloric supplementation
during the latter pregnancy was lower than during the preceding pregnancy, the
birth weight of the latter baby was also lower than the birth weight of the
preceding baby. When the caloric supplementation during the latter pregnancy
was higher than that during the preceding pregnancy, the latter newborn was
heavier than the preceding one. The intermediate group is composed of siblings
in which the increment in caloric supplementation during the latter pregnancy
was between 100 and 20,000 calories. The difference in birth weight between

both babies is close to zero and, therefore, intermediate between the extreme groups.

In summary: When a mother in our sample consumed more in one pregnancy than in another, there was a significant tendency for the baby of that pregnancy to be heavier at birth. We therefore conclude that caloric supplementation during pregnancy caused the observed decrease of the proportion of small babies in our study population.

EFFECT OF MATERNAL NUTRITION ON INFANT GROWTH

Maternal malnutrition during pregnancy and lactation has been implicated as one of several environmental factors contributing to postnatal growth retardation. Maternal nutrition is associated with the output of breast milk during lactation (2, 23, 26, 32, 46, 52, 58), which in turn is an important determinant of early postnatal growth in breast-fed infants (2, 24, 29, 31). This observation led us to postulate a causal relationship between maternal nutrition and the infant's physical growth. However, the design and data analyses of most of the published reports do not allow for assessment of a causal relationship between maternal nutrition and infant growth. Data from the INCAP study supports the hypothesis of a causal relationship between maternal nutrition and infant growth (35, 39, 40).

Table 11–7 shows the mean attained growth in weight and height to 6 months of age for each of three categories of cumulative maternal caloric supplementation since conception. Also included in this table are the t and P values for the differences between high and low supplementation groups. The existence of a consistent trend for children in the high category to be heavier and taller than children in the low category is apparent in these data.

The associations found between food supplementation and infant growth could, however, be due to factors other than supplementation. Such possible confounding factors must be excluded to claim a nutritional effect. For example, the mothers and children who attended the supplementation centers may have had better home diets or were healthier than subjects who did not attend the centers. However, analyses indicate that the association found between supplemented calories and infant growth is not explained by maternal and infant diet, family socioeconomic status, maternal and child morbidity, gestational age, or maternal anthropometric and obstetric characteristics.

The possibility also exists that sample mothers with heavier babies were those who tended to collaborate with the program. If this were the case, the observed association between caloric supplementation and growth would be artifactual. To explore the possibility that some constant maternal factor might be responsible for both the high consumption of food supplement and better growth, we again studied consecutive siblings of the same mother. Table 11–8 indicates the difference in weight for 111 pairs of siblings divided into three groups according to the differences between both siblings.

It is evident that there is an association between differences in cumulative

Table 11–7 ATTAINED WEIGHT AND HEIGHT FOR THREE CATEGORIES OF CUMULATIVE
CALORIC SUPPLEMENTATION SINCE CONCEPTION

Age (mos)		Weight (kg)			t Test (low–high)	Height (cm)			t Test (high–low)
		Low	Intermediate	High		Low	Intermediate	High	
3	Mean	5.21	5.29	5.41	2.46*	56.5	56.6	57.4	3.14*
	N	155	168	105		155	169	105	
6	Mean	6.58	6.61	6.81	1.99†	62.1	62.1	62.7	1.92
	N	133	217	97		134	217	96	

*P < 0.01.
†P < 0.05.

Table 11–8. RELATIONSHIP BETWEEN DIFFERENCES IN CUMULATIVE MATERNAL CALORIC SUP-
PLEMENTATION SINCE CONCEPTION AND DIFFERENCES IN ATTAINED WEIGHT AT
6 MONTHS OF AGE FOR TWO CONSECUTIVE SIBLINGS (LATTER MINUS PRECEDING
CHILD)

Differences in caloric supplementation	Differences in infant weight (mean ± SD) (g)	N
−40,000 – 0 cal	−247 ± 788	39
100 – 20,000 cal	−107 ± 861	34
20,100 – 120,000 cal	280 ± 920	38

t Test (high–low) = 2.70; P < .01.

caloric supplementation of the pregnant and lactating mother up to 6 months
after birth and differences in attained weight between siblings. Similar results
have been found with attained height and with increments in weight and height
from 0 to 6 months of age. The most suitable interpretation of these results is
that food supplementation of both the pregnant and lactating mother caused an
improvement of the infant's growth up to 6 months of age.

EFFECT OF MATERNAL NUTRITION ON MENTAL DEVELOPMENT

BIRTH WEIGHT AND MENTAL DEVELOPMENT

It has been reported that low birth weight is associated with deficits in mental
performance (5, 8). Although many published studies ignore potentially confounding factors, those that have considered such variables support the conclusion that there is an association between low birth weight and poor mental
performance (13–15, 21, 51, 53, 59, 60). Recently, we presented data which
supports the conclusion that birth weight and psychomotor performance during
the first months of life are associated (36).

Our sample includes 405 live newborns with birth weight data. Some of these
newborns were tested by the Brazelton Assessment Scale within the first 2
weeks of life. This scale consists of 44 items which assess arousal state, irritabil-

ity, motor capabilities, reaction to external stimuli, and neonatal reflexes. These 44 items were grouped into 11 summary variables of which the four with significant test–retest reliability have been analyzed. The Composite Infant Scale (CIS) was administered at 6 months of age and consisted of 91 items drawn from four widely used scales assessing psychomotor development in infancy, the Bayley, Catell, Merrill-Palmer, and Gesell scales. The 91 items comprising the scale were grouped into two subscales, mental and motor, each of which has test–retest reliability above .88.

Table 11–9 shows the correlation coefficients between birth weight and performance on the Brazelton and CIS Scales.

Birth weight is clearly associated with performance on three of the four Brazelton variables: habituation, motor fitness, and tremors and startles. The correlation between birth weight and the motor subscale of the CIS was also significant. Furthermore, the associations between birth weight and the other performance variables, although nonsignificant, were in the expected direction.

To examine alternative explanations, we measured approximately 50 factors which could be confounding or causal factors in the observed associations between birth weight and performance. After controlling for each of these variables, the association between birth weight and CIS motor performance remained significant.

We also explored differences between siblings in order to determine whether the relationship between birth weight and psychomotor performance was due to differences between mothers related to both birth weight and performance of their infants. In our sample we have 65 pairs of consecutive siblings on whom we have both birth weight and 6 months CIS data. The significant relationship observed in the entire sample between birth weight and performance on the motor subscale was replicated with this sibling sample ($r = .266$, $P < .05$). Therefore, the association between birth weight and psychomotor performance is consistent in the whole population and between siblings.

A reasonable interpretation of these results is that birth weight is related to psychomotor development during the first half year of life in these villages.

CALORIC SUPPLEMENTATION AND MENTAL DEVELOPMENT

Available data on psychologic test performance are sufficient to address the question of the relationship between food supplementation and infant psychologic test performance from birth to 6 months of age (34, 35). The association

Table 11–9. ASSOCIATION OF PSYCHOLOGIC TEST PERFORMANCE WITH BIRTH WEIGHT

Brazelton variables				CIS	
Motor fitness (N=144)	Tremors & startles (N=145)	Habituation (N=141)	Alertness (N=145)	Mental (N=352)	Motor (N=352)
0.28*	−0.17†	0.27*	0.12	0.10	0.16*

*$P < 0.01$.
†$P < 0.05$.

between infant mental test performance and supplement ingestion is presented in Table 11–10.

Turning first to the results of evaluation of the infant shortly after birth, we note that although food supplementation during gestation was associated with higher birth weight, performance on the Brazelton Neonatal Evaluation Scale was not affected. The two Brazelton variables reported here are derived from clusters of items that appeared together in factor analyses of all test items. BB1 includes the negative signs of tonus, motor maturity, vigor, pull to sit, visual following, trembling, and interest in the examiner. BG1 is to some degree the

Table 11–10. PSYCHOLOGIC TEST PERFORMANCE BY THREE CATEGORIES OF CUMULATIVE MATERNAL CALORIC SUPPLEMENTATION DURING PREGNANCY AND LACTATION

Psychologic test score		Level of maternal caloric supplementation			
		Low	Intermediate	High	F
Brazelton Neonatal Assessment					
BB1	Mean	39.69	40.00	39.54	0.02
	N	42	32	83	
BG1	Mean	38.83	36.00	39.05	0.66
	N	42	32	83	
Composite Infant Scale (6 mos)					
Mental scale	Mean	73.8	76.3	77.8	2.87*
	N	150	221	101	
Motor scale	Mean	70.0	70.6	72.7	1.13
	N	150	221	101	

*$P < 0.05$.

Table 11–11. ASSOCIATION OF PSYCHOLOGIC TEST PERFORMANCE WITH SUPPLEMENT INGESTION

Test	I. Supplement ingested during pregnancy	II. Total supplement ingested to time of testing	III. Total Supplement ingested to time of testing (II). Controlling for supplement ingested during pregnancy (I)	IV. Supplement ingested during pregnancy (I). Controlling for postnatal supplement ingested to time of testing (II)
Boys				
Composite Infant Scale (6 mos) mental scale	.11	.04	−.07	.13*
Girls				
Composite Infant Scale (6 mos) mental scale	.13*	.01	−.018†	.15*

*$P < 0.05$.
†$P < 0.01$.

opposite of BB1; it includes the positive signs of vigor, visual following, social interest in the examiner, and motor maturity.

Table 11–10 also reports results for the Composite Infant Scale at 6 months of age. At this age, only the mental scale is significantly associated with supplement ingestion.

There were relatively few sex differences with respect to the impact of food supplementation on psychologic test performance in this age range. In general, performances of boys and girls were comparable, and they responded similarly to food supplementation.

Table 11–11 presents data on the effects of the timing of supplement ingestion on psychologic test performance. Presented are correlations and partial correlations of Composite Infant Scale mental scores at 6 months with supplement ingestion. Not only are the correlations between gestational supplementation and test performance at 6 months of age significant, but once gestational supplementation is partialled out of the correlations between total cumulative supplementation and test score association, virtually no relationship remains between later cumulative supplementation and test performance. On the other hand, the effect of prenatal supplement and subsequent test performance is unaffected by controlling for later supplementation. Thus, as the previous analyses indicated, pregnancy is the crucial period for supplementation as far as the 6 months psychologic test performance is concerned.

The design of the present study, like those of many large-scale intervention studies, does not eliminate completely the possibility of confounding and subsequent misinterpretation of results. To avoid this possibility, we conducted a series of detailed analyses exploring various alternative interpretations of the results presented here. The first is the study of associations between supplement and psychologic test performance with the same mother from child to child. As in the case of birth weight and infant growth, these analyses show statistically significant relationships. In other words, even within the same family greater maternal supplement ingestion during one pregnancy is associated with superior test performance of that child.

EFFECT OF MATERNAL NUTRITION ON INFANT MORTALITY

Low birth weight is well established as an antecedent of excessive mortality in infants. Data from the United States (3, 9) and England (6) indicate that infant death rates rise dramatically among newborns weighing 2500 g or less. Developing countries present a high incidence of low-birth-weight babies, which have a higher risk of death (57) and are more susceptible to infectious diseases (47). Within our sample, infant mortality in babies of birth weight of 2.5 kg or less is nearly two times as much as that found in babies of birth weight greater than 2.5 kg (30, 39).

We have also found that infant mortality decreases as the level of maternal supplementation during pregnancy and lactation increases (Table 11–12).

Table 11–12 reports the association between caloric supplementation and

Table 11–12. INFANT MORTALITY BY THREE CATEGORIES OF CUMULATIVE MATERNAL CA-
LORIC SUPPLEMENTATION DURING PREGNANCY AND LACTATION

| | Level of cumulative maternal caloric supplementation | | |
	Low	Intermediate	High
Infant deaths	25	12	7
Number of infants	274	258	121
Infant death rate/1000	91.24	46.51	57.85

stillbirths and infant deaths during the first year of life. The proportion of deaths in the lower supplemented group was greater than in the intermediate and high groups. The magnitude of the difference is such that the risk of dying during the first year of life in the highly supplemented group is almost two thirds of that observed in the low supplemented group. These results indicate that child mortality decreases as the level of maternal supplementation increases.

EFFECT OF MATERNAL NUTRITION ON BIRTHSPACING

Several authors have postulated that malnutrition lowers the reproductive capacity of populations (12, 25, 27, 55). Some experimental evidence supports the plausibility of the above hypothesis. Chavez and Martinez (10), working with a small sample of Mexican women, report findings that suggest that one of the effects of supplementing the diet of pregnant and lactating women is to significantly reduce the duration of postpartum amenorrhea in nursing women. It was reported that mothers receiving food supplementation began menstruating at 7.5 months after delivery compared to control mothers, who began menstruating 14 months after giving birth.

The possibility that nutrition is related to fecundity is also given some support by the findings of Lev-Ran (44), who reported cases of secondary amenorrhea in young normal women following strict weight reduction diets. Similarly, the prevalence of amenorrhea has been reported to increase during times of severe food shortage and famine (1, 54).

Thus, differing lines of evidence suggest that nutrition may be an important determinant of human fecundity. While this proposition seems reasonable, there is at present a lack of direct empirical data to support it. One of the many areas explored in the longitudinal study has been the interrelationship between lactation, menstruation, and pregnancy (17–19). Since data have been collected prospectively (all the families are visited every 14 days), reliable information has been obtained in the areas of total birth interval, length of postpartum amenorrhea, length of menstruating interval, duration of lactation, outcome of the previous delivery, and survival of the last child born.

The median duration of lactation in the study communities is 18 months and of postpartum amenorrhea 14 months (means are 17 and 14 months, respectively). The two variables are highly associated, the correlation coefficient being .63 (334 cases, $P < .01$). In these analyses we have excluded cases of stillbirth or death in the first year of life. The median duration of postpartum amenorrhea in nursing women in our study is comparable to those reported in rural populations. Potter *et al.* (50), in a prospective study in India, reported a median of 11 months; Berman *et al.* (4), in a study on Eskimo women, reported a median of 10 months; and Chen *et al.* (12), in a study in Bangladesh reported a median of 13 months.

Data from the longitudinal study reveal a negative association between indicators of past and present nutritional status of the mother such as weight, height, head and arm circumference, and duration of postpartum amenorrhea, indicating that the better the nutritional status of the mother, the shorter the postpartum amenorrhea. A negative association was also found between home caloric intake and length of amenorrhea. Other variables, such as parity, previous birth interval, and age of the mother, were found to be positively correlated with duration of postpartum amenorrhea.

The longitudinal study data indicate a negative association between caloric supplementation ingested during pregnancy and duration of postpartum amenorrhea in both atole and fresco villages. However, in atole villages (where supplementation consisted of carbohydrates, proteins, and fat) this correlation is statistically significant ($r = -.199$, $P < .01$, $N = 171$), whereas in fresco villages (where supplementation consisted of carbohydrates only, in lesser concentrations than in atole villages) it is not. Significant differences in duration of postpartum amenorrhea between atole and fresco villages have not been found.

Another way of looking at these data consists of comparing the high-calorie and low-calorie supplemented groups within types of villages (atole versus fresco), as shown in Figure 11–1.

Two categories of supplementation were constructed: more than 20,000 calories during pregnancy, and 20,000 calories or less. Our data indicate that the high-calorie supplemented group in the atole villages had a significantly shorter duration of postpartum amenorrhea than the low-calorie supplemented group (*t* test, $P < .05$). Within fresco villages this difference, though in the expected direction, was not statistically significant. It should be noted that the reduction in the length of amenorrhea in the highly supplemented groups cannot be attributed to a reduction in the duration of lactation between the two groups. As shown in Figure 11–1, high and low supplemented groups exhibited virtually identical lactation intervals. These results indicate that in atole and in fresco villages the interval of lactation and menstruation (duration of lactation minus the length of postpartum amenorrhea) was longer in the high supplemented group than in the low supplemented group. This interval was positively associated with the amount of supplementation during pregnancy, significantly in atole villages ($P < .05$) and nonsignificantly in fresco villages. Furthermore, preliminary analyses showed that the amount of protein-calorie supplementation ingested by the mother during lactation was negatively associated not only with the duration of postpartum amenorrhea but also with the duration of the menstruating interval.

Table 11–13 shows the mean duration of lactation and postpartum amenorrhea for each of the three categories of cumulative calorie supplementation of sample pregnant and lactating mothers up to 6 months postpartum. Low and

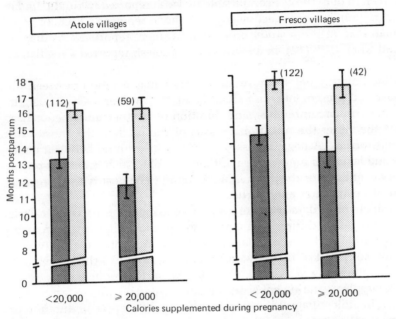

Fig. 11–1. Relationship between caloric supplementation during pregnancy and duration of postpartum amenorrhea *(hatched columns)* and lactation *(dotted columns)* in atole and fresco villages. The columns are of mean values, and the standard error is indicated by the vertical lines. Number of women studied is in parentheses.

Table 11–13. DURATION OF LACTATION AND POSTPARTUM AMENORRHEA

| | Level of cumulative maternal caloric supplementation | | | |
	Low	Intermediate	High	*t* Test (high–low)
Duration of lactation (mos)	18.40	17.98	17.61	1.15
Duration of postpartum amenorrhea (mos)	14.93	13.90	12.83	2.22*
Number of mothers	94	164	76	

*$P < 0.05$.

high supplemented groups showed nearly identical durations of lactation. On the other hand, the existence of a consistent trend for mothers in the intermediate and high supplementation categories to have a shorter postpartum amenorrhea than mothers in the low category is apparent in these data.

These results give partial support to the hypothesis that improvement of maternal nutrition is associated with a decrease in the duration of postpartum amenorrhea, and that this may increase the probability of a shorter birth interval. Though suggestive, these results suffer from weakness. No control was exerted over several possible sources of errors, including self-selection, cooperation, and frequency of sucking. Concerning the latter, it has been reported that the frequency of sucking and the amount of food supplemented to the infant during the first year of life may be important determinants of the duration of postpartum amenorrhea. It has also been suggested that food supplementation during lactation may diminish the sucking reflex and may also discourage lactation through a "substitution" effect, thereby shortening the period of postpartum amenorrhea (11).

The data presented suggest that poor nutrition and prolonged lactation lengthen the period of postpartum amenorrhea and, consequently, decrease reproductive capacity. Given that poor nutrition and prolonged lactation are characteristics of poor societies in developing nations, it is tempting to infer that fecundity and, consequently, fertility would be much higher in these areas were it not for these factors.

Despite the fact that poor nutritional status probably reduces the length of the infertile period following birth during which ovulation does not occur, it is difficult to estimate what the outcome of a nutrition program would be. It is easy of course to predict a population increase from the results presented and cited above. However, bettering nutritional status may in fact result in unchanged or lowered fecundity for the following reasons. Better maternal nutrition is associated with a longer period of lactation (17). Further, better nutrition may reduce infant mortality (39) and should, therefore, prolong lactation in cases where a death would have occurred. The increase in the length of lactation might then increase the length of the period of postpartum amenorrhea, compensating therefore the effect of nutrition per se on postpartum amenorrhea.

CONCLUSION

Information obtained from the published reports as well as from our own data leads us to believe that an improvement in the nutritional status of pregnant and lactating women is associated with a significant decrease in the prevalence of physical growth retardation up to 6 months of age and also of infant mortality. Nutrition also appears to be associated with psychologic test performance and birthspacing.

REFERENCES

1. Antonov AN: Children born during the siege of Leningrad in 1942. J Pediatr 30:250, 1947
2. Bailey KV: Quantity and composition of breast milk in some New Guinean populations. J Trop Pediatr 11:35, 1965
3. Bergner L, Susser M: Low birthweight and prenatal nutrition: an interpretative review. Pediatrics 46:946, 1970
4. Berman ML, Hanson K, Hellman I: Effect of breast-feeding on postpartum menstruation, ovulation and pregnancy in Alaskan Eskimos. Am J Obstet Gynecol 114:524, 1972

5. Birch HG, Gussow JD: Disadvantaged Children. New York, Harcourt, Brace & World, 1970
6. Brinblecombe F, Ashford J: Significance of low birthweight in perinatal mortality: a study of variations within England and Wales. Br J Prev Soc Med 22:27, 1968
7. Burke BS, Beal VA, Kirkwood SB, Stuart HC: The influence of nutrition during pregnancy upon the condition of the infant at birth. J Nutr 26:569, 1943
8. Caputo DV, Mandell W: Consequences of low birthweight. Dev Psychol 3:363, 1970
9. Chase HC: Infant mortality and weight at birth: 1960. United States cohort. Am J Public Health 59:1618, 1969
10. Chavez A, Martinez C: Nutrition and development of infants from poor rural areas. III. Maternal nutrition and its consequences on fertility. Nutr Rep Int 7:1, 1973
11. Chen LC: Nutrition and fertility. Lancet 1:47, 1973
12. Chen LC, Ahmed S, Gesche M, Mosley WH: A prospective study of birth interval dynamics in rural Bangladesh. Pop Studies 28(2):277, 1974
13. Churchill JA: The relationship between intelligence and birthweight in twins. Neurology (Minneap) 15:341, 1965
14. Dann M, Levine SZ, New EV: The development of prematurely born children with birthweights or minimal postnatal weights of 1000 grams or less. Pediatrics 22:1037, 1958
15. Dann M, Levine SZ, New EV: A long-term follow-up of small premature infants. Pediatrics 33:945, 1964
16. DDH/INCAP: Nutricion, crecimiento y desarrollo. Bol Of Sanit Panam 78:38, 1975
17. Delgado H, Habicht JP, Lechtig A, Klein RE, Yarbrough C, Martorell R: Prenatal nutrition. Paper presented at the Symposium on "Current Concepts in Nutrition: Nutrition in the Life Cycle". Los Angeles, University of Southern California, 1973
18. Delgado H, Lechtig A, Martorell R, Yarbrough C, Klein RE: Efectos de la nutrición materna sobre la duración de la lactancia y de la amenorrhea post-parto. Paper presented at the 2do Congreso Peruano de Nutricion, Trujillo, Peru, 1975
19. Delgado H., Lechtig A., Yarbrough C., Martorell R., Klein R.E.: Effect of improved nutrition on the duration of post-partum amenorrhea in moderate malnourished populations. In: *Xth International Congress of Nutrition,* (Abstract No. 3325). Kyoto, Japan, 1975, p. 182.
20. Dieckman WJ, Adain FL, Michael H, Kiamen S, Dunkle F, Arthur B, Costin M, Campbell A, Winsley AC, Lorang E: Calcium, phosphorus, iron and nitrogen balance in pregnant women. Am J Obstet Gynecol 47:357, 1944
21. Douglas JWB: Mental ability and school achievement of premature children at eight years of age. Br Med J 1:1210, 1956
22. Ebbs J, Tisdall FF, Scott WA: The influence of prenatal diet on the mother and child. J Nutr 22:515, 1941
23. Edozien JC: Malnutrition in Africa—need and basis for action. Bibl Nutr Dieta 14:64, 1970
24. Fomon SJ, Thomas LN, Filer LJ, Ziegler EE, Leonard MT: Food consumption and growth of normal infants fed milk-based formulas. Acta Paediatr Scand 223:3, 1971
25. Frisch RE: Demographic implications of the biological determinants of female fecundity. Paper presented at the annual meeting of the Population Association of America, New York, 1974
26. Gopalan C: Effect of protein supplementation and some so-called galactogogues on lactation of poor Indian women. Indian J Med Res 46:317, 1958
27. Gopalan C, Naidu AN: Nutrition and fertility. Lancet 2:1077, 1972
28. Gruenwald P, Funakawa H, Mitani S, Nishimura T, Takeuchi S: Influence of environmental factors on foetal growth in man. Lancet 1:1026, 1967
29. Gunther M, Stanier JE: The volume and composition of human milk. Spec Rep Ser Med Res Counc 275:379, 1951
30. Habicht JP, Lechtig A, Yarbrough C, Delgado H, Klein RE: The effect of malnutrition during pregnancy on survival of the newborn. Testimony presented at the hearing

of the Select Committee on Nutrition and Human Needs. Washington DC, US Senate, June 5, 1973

31. Hytten FE: Clinical and chemical studies in human lactation. VII. The effect of differences in yield and composition of milk on the infants weight gain and the duration of breast feeding. Br Med J 1:1410, 1954

32. Jansen AAJ, Luyken R, Malcolm SH, Willems JJ: Quantity and composition of breast milk in Biak Island. Trop Geogr Med 12:138, 1960

33. Klein RE, Habicht JP, Yarbrough C: Some methodological problems in field studies of nutrition and intelligence. In Kallen DJ (ed): Nutrition, Development and Social Behavior. Washington DC, US Government Printing Office, DHEW Pub No. (NIH) 73–242, 1973, pp 61–75

34. Klein R.E., Irwin M.H., Engle P.L., Yarbrough C.: Malnutrition and mental development in rural Guatemala: an applied cross-cultural research study. In: N. Warren (ed.): *Advances in Cross-Cultural Psychology*, New York: Academic Press, 1976, in press.

35. Klein R.E., *et al.*: Effect of maternal nutrition on fetal growth and infant development. *Pan American Sanitary Bureau Bulletin*, 1976, in press.

36. Lasky RE, Lechtig A, Delgado H, Klein RE, Engle P, Yarbrough C, Martorell R: Birth weight and psychomotor performance in rural Guatemala. Am J Dis Child 129:566, 1975

37. Lechtig A, Delgado H, Lasky RE, Klein RE, Engle PL, Yarbrough C, Habicht JP: Maternal nutrition and fetal growth in developing societies. Socioeconomic factors. Am J Dis Child 129:434, 1975

38. Lechtig A, Delgado H, Lasky RE, Yarbrough C, Klein RE, Habicht JP, Béhar M: Maternal nutrition and fetal growth in developing countries. Am J Dis Child 129:553, 1975

39. Lechtig A., Delgado H., Lasky R.E., Yarbrough C., Martorell R., Habicht J-P. & Klein R.E.: Effect of improved nutrition during pregnancy and lactation on developmental retardation and infant mortality. In: P. L. White & N. Selvey, (eds.): *Proceedings of the Western Hemisphere Nutrition Congress IV, 1974*, Acton, Mass.: Publishing Sciences Group Inc., 1975, pp. 117–125

40. Lechtig A, Delgado H, Martorell R, Yarbrough C, Klein RE: Effect of improved nutrition since conception on growth retardation up to three years of age and on infant mortality. In Xth Int Congr Nutr (abstr no. 342). Kyoto, Japan, 1975, p 34

41. Lechtig A, Habicht JP, de Leon E, Guzmán G, Flores M: Influencia de la nutrición materna sobre el crecimiento fetal en poblaciones rurales de Guatemala. 1. Aspectos dietéticos. Arch Latinoam Nutr 22:101, 1972

42. Lechtig A, Habicht JP, Delgado H, Klein RE, Yarbrough C, Martorell R: Effect of food supplementation during pregnancy on birthweight. Pediatrics 56:508, 1975

43. Lechtig A., Yarbrough C., Delgado H., Habicht J-P., Martorell R., & Klein R.E.: Influence of maternal nutrition on birth weight. *American Journal of Clinical Nutrition, 28*: 1223, 1975.

44. Lev–Ran A: Secondary amenorrhea resulting from uncontrolled weight-reducing diets. Fertil Steril 25:459, 1974

45. Lindblad BS, Rahimtoola R: A pilot study of the quality of human milk in a lower socio-economic group in Karachi, Pakistan. Acta Paediatr Scand 63:125, 1974

46. Lyengar L: Effect of dietary supplements on birth weight of infants. In 1st Asian Congr Nutr. Abstracts, Symposia, Special Reports, Research Communications. Hyderabad, India, 20 Kamal Printers, 1971, p 126

47. Mata L, Urrutia JJ, Behar M: Infección en la mujer embarazada y en los productos de la concepcion. Arch Latinoam Nutr 24:15, 1974

48. McGanity WJ, Cannon RO, Bridgforth EB, Martin MP, Denson PM, Newbill JA, McClellan GS, Christie A, Peterson CJ, Darby WJ: The Vanderbilt Cooperative study of maternal and infant nutrition. VI. Relationship of obstetric performance to nutrition. Am J Obstet Gynecol 67:501, 1954

49. Niswander KL: The women and their pregnancies. Washington DC, US Department of Health, Education and Welfare, Pub No. (NIH) 73–379, 1972
50. Potter RG, New ML, Wyon JB, Gordon JE: Applications of field studies to research on the physiology of human reproduction: lactation and its effects on birth intervals in eleven Punjab Villages, India. J Chronic Dis 18:1125, 1965
51. Rabinovitch MS, Bibace R, Caplan H: Sequelae of prematurity: psychological test findings. Can Med Assoc J 84:822, 1961
52. Rao KS, Swaminathan MC, Swarup S, Pathwardhan VN: Protein malnutrition in South India. Bull WHO 20:603, 1959
53. Robinson NM, Robinson HB: A follow-up study of children of low birth weight and control children at school age. Pediatrics 35:425, 1965
54. Smith CA: Effects of maternal undernutrition upon the newborn infant in Holland (1944–45). J Pediatr 30:229, 1947
55. Solien de González N: Lactation and pregnancy: a hypothesis. Am Anthropol 66:873, 1964
56. Thomson AM: Diet in pregnancy. 3. Diet in relation to the course and outcome of pregnancy. Br J Nutr 13:509, 1959
57. Van den Berg B, Yerushalmy J: The relationship of the rate of intrauterine growth of infants of low birthweight to mortality, morbidity and congenital anomalies. J Pediatr 69:531, 1966
58. Venkatachalam PS: Study of the Diet, Nutrition and Health of the People of the Chimbut Area. (Monograph No. 4). New Guinea, Department of Public Health, Government of Papua, 1962
59. Wiener G: Psychologic correlates of premature birth: a review. J Nerv Ment Dis 134:129, 1962
60. Wiener G, Rider RV, Oppel WC, Harper PA: Correlates of low birthweight: psychological status at eight to ten years of age. Pediatr Res 2:110, 1968

Chapter 12

Relationship of Nutrition to Lactation and Newborn Development

Lloyd J. Filer, Jr.

THE PRACTICE OF BREAST-FEEDING

The 1970s has seen a renewed interest in the practice of breast-feeding in the United States. Twenty-five years ago, 3 women in 10 elected to breast-feed their infant at the time of their hospital discharge. This ratio has now risen to 4 in 10. The practice of breast-feeding, however, is not uniform throughout the United States. On a percentage basis, eastern states, both north and south, have had fewer women involved in breast-feeding than the mountain or western states. This difference amounts to a factor of two. In addition to greater numbers of women breast-feeding in the 1970s, it is also evident that more women are breast-feeding their infants for longer periods of time. According to Martinez, the percentage of infants being breast-fed to 4 months of age in 1974 is 1.6 times greater than the percentage of 4-month-old infants breast-fed in 1972 (16) (Table 12–1). These observations of Martinez are highly significant in view of the study by Sloper and coworkers demonstrating that while it was possible to increase the number of infants breast-fed at the time of hospital discharge, no greater percentage of infants was being breast-fed at 2 months of age (28). The commitment to breast-feeding by many of the mothers in this study was short-lived.

It is difficult to assign reasons for the sharp decline in the practice of breast-feeding in the United States, and it is equally difficult to understand the forces that have produced a turnaround or increase in breast-feeding. One factor which may contribute to the problem is the number of mothers in the labor force. In 1940, 25% of the labor force of the United States was female and 10% of these women were mothers. By 1970, the labor force was 40% female and 40% of these women were mothers (24). In three decades the number of mothers in the labor force had increased sevenfold. Working mothers frequently find it difficult to nurse an infant. However, many of the social changes currently occurring in the United States directly or indirectly support the practice of breast-feeding.

Both developed and developing countries are experiencing trends away from breast-feeding. As yet, data showing that these trends have slowed or reversed themselves in countries other than the United States are not available although

Table 12–1. PERCENT OF BREAST-FED INFANTS IN THE UNITED STATES

Year	Age of infant (mos)			
	3	4	5	6
1972	10	10	5	5
1974	18	16	14	7

considerable effort is being made to achieve this objective. The Protein Advisory Group of the United Nations is trying desperately to stem the move away from breast-feeding that is occurring in developing countries (21, 22). In their efforts to do so, they have solicited the support of the physician, nurse, health educator, respective national and local governments, and members of the food industry. If we understood the "why" in the United States, this possibly could be applied to the world at large.

The most systematic approach to understanding the factors that influence breast-feeding may come out of the Swedish experience. The percent of breast-fed infants in Sweden has decreased precipitously since World War II (27). This alarming state of affairs has stimulated the Swedish government and members of the health professions to find means to increase the practice of breast-feeding in Sweden.

While we certainly do not understand the societal changes that are influencing attitudes toward breast-feeding, we should not lose sight of the fact that the structural function of the human breast has not changed dramatically in the last 100 years (19). Those best equipped to understand how cultural patterns are modified should be aware of changes in the practice of breast-feeding and provide rational answers for the trend.

DIET AND COMPOSITION OF HUMAN MILK

FATS AND FATTY ACIDS

Alterations in maternal diet can influence the concentration of some components of breast milk. Fatty acid patterns of human milk can be changed by modifying energy intake and the fatty acid composition of dietary fat (9). Lactating women fed a diet rich in polyunsaturated fats such as corn or soybean oil will produce milk with an increased content of polyunsaturated fats. Such dietary changes are without effect on volume of milk produced or its total fat content. With caloric restriction the fatty acid composition of human milk resembles that of depot fat. This signifies fat mobilization in response to a reduced energy intake. An increase in energy intake as carbohydrate will result in an increase in content of lauric and myristic acids. This change in composition of human milk is of interest in view of the report by Sinclair and Crawford of increased mortality and reduced body size and brain cell number among rats nourished by dams whose milk contains a high content of short and medium chain fatty acids (26).

Human milk provides 50% of total energy (kilocalories) in the form of a readily absorbed or digestible fat. This high caloric density feeding enables the newborn to obtain its energy requirements in a volume of feeding that its gut can manage. The high coefficient of absorption of human milk fat (95%) is a function of the specificity of its triglyceride structure (Table 12–2). Dietary fats with a high content of triglycerides having a predominance of palmitic acid in the two or β-position of the glycerol molecule are readily absorbed (5). Biosynthesis of stereospecific triglycerides is species dependent and cannot be modified through dietary means. Thus the fatty acid pattern but not the triglyceride structure of human milk fat can be modified by maternal diet.

PROTEIN AND AMINO ACIDS

Protein content of human milk is not reduced in mothers consuming a diet low in protein or poor in protein quality. A recent study by Lindblad and Rahimtoola on the quality of human milk collected from a low socioeconomic group in Karachi, Pakistan, confirms the constancy of protein content (14). When the amino acid content of these milk samples was compared to milk from healthy well-nourished mothers, the content of two essential amino acids, lysine and methionine, was found to be reduced. This could imply a reduction in nutritional quality of milk protein. Within very wide limits it seems reasonable to conclude that lactation can be subsidized from maternal tissues as long as reserves are available.

Protein content of human milk does decrease during the first 6 months of lactation; however, from 6 to 24 months of lactation the protein content of milk remains relatively constant.

Data on the composition of milk of 17 healthy nursing women living in Iowa

Table 12–2. TRIGLYCERIDE STRUCTURE AND ABSORPTION OF DIETARY FAT

Fat	C_{16} in two position (%)	Absorption (%)
Human	68	96
Lard	85	95
Randomized lard	34	72
Butterfat	43	61

Table 12–3. AVERAGE COMPOSITION OF HUMAN MILK

Stage of lactation (days)	Total solids (g/liter)	Protein (g/liter)	Ca (mg/liter)	P (mg/liter)	Mg (mg/liter)	Na (mg/liter)	K (mg/liter)	Zn (mg/liter)
14	126.5	15.4	278	188	30	204	421	3.7
28	127.6	13.8	261	169	28	161	347	2.6
42	122.7	12.6	255	151	28	151	367	2.2
56	116.1	10.9	266	150	31	135	374	2.0
84	116.6	10.2	247	130	30	125	343	2.0
112	127.7	8.7	236	132	32	120	296	1.1

City are summarized in Table 12–3 (7). A decrease in protein, calcium, phosphorus, sodium, potassium, and zinc concentrations during 4 months of lactation is apparent. Magnesium concentration does not change. Similar results have been reported by Ko for lactating Korean women followed in a large private pediatric clinic in Seoul (12).

We have measured free amino acid concentrations in plasma and breast milk of 10 women with established lactation following a single loading dose of lactose or monosodium glutamate (29). Each compound was administered in the fasting state at a level of 100 mg/kg body weight. An increase in plasma concentration of glutamic acid, glutamine, aspartic acid, and alanine was noted; however, no detectable change occurred in the concentration of these free amino acids in breast milk samples collected concurrently over a period of 12 hours.

CALCIUM

There is no evidence that the calcium content of human milk can be influenced by varying the calcium content of the diet. According to Liu and coworkers, poorly fed Chinese mothers with histories of severe calcium depletion produce milk with normal calcium levels (15). Using the technique of scanning transmission, Atkinson and West have shown that healthy lactating women mobilize about 2.2% of femoral bone mineral in 100 days (1). If one assumes that this loss applies to the total skeleton or body pool of calcium, which approximates 1.2 kg, the daily mobilization of calcium can be estimated as 250 mg.

TRACE ELEMENTS

The iron, copper, and fluoride content of human milk is not altered by administration of these trace elements to lactating women. Indeed, the total fluorine content of human milk from mothers using fluoridated drinking water does not differ from that of mothers using nonfluoridated water (3).

Since epidemiologic studies indicate that an increase in dietary selenium may accentuate dental caries, Shearer and Hadjimarkos have measured the selenium content of a large number of human milk samples collected in the United States (25). While the results tend to support the hypothesis that lactating women residing in areas of the country where forage crops are high in selenium produce milk high in selenium, the data are far from conclusive (Table 12–4).

We have recently measured the mercury content of mature human milk samples collected in Iowa City (23). Detectable mercury levels were found in 14 of 32 samples. Assuming values below the limit of detection to be zero, mean concentration was 0.96 parts/billion. These results are compatible with our observations on mercury concentrations in the placenta and maternal and cord blood, reflecting the relatively low mercury exposure of a rural population.

Studies on the iron and fluoride content of human milk should be of interest to those responsible for well child care; however, it should be recognized that the LaLeche League does not advocate administration of iron and fluoride to breast-fed infants.

VITAMINS

Administration of fat-soluble vitamins A, D, and E to lactating women does not raise the level of these vitamins in milk. The vitamin D content of human milk is so low that breast-fed infants do not obtain their recommended daily requirement and have been observed to develop rickets. The situation with respect to the water-soluble vitamins is entirely different. Levels of these vitamins in breast milk reflect dietary intake. Following large oral doses of water-soluble vitamins, marked but transient increases in their concentration occurs in milk. The relationship between diet and water-soluble vitamin content of human milk is best illustrated by reports of death from beriberi of Burmese infants nursed by mothers with beriberi.

For reasons stated in the section on trace elements and vitamins, breast-fed infants should receive a supplement of iron, fluoride, and vitamin D.

DIET FOR THE NURSING MOTHER

The Food and Nutrition Board Committee on Recommended Daily Dietary Allowances considers the optimal diet for the lactating woman a diet which supplies somewhat more of each nutrient, with the exception of vitamin D, than that recommended for the nonpregnant female (Table 12–5). Major increases are seen for energy intake, i.e., an additional 500 kcal/day and protein an additional 20 g/day (18).

Approximately 900 kcal are required for the production of 1 liter of milk. During a normal pregnancy, women store 2–4 kg of body fat which can be mobilized to supply a portion of the additional energy for lactation. Storage fat will provide 200–300 kcal/day during a lactation period approximating 100 days, i.e., one-third the energy cost to produce 850 ml milk/day. On this basis an additional 500 kcals/day should be supplied during the first 3 months of lactation to permit readjustment of maternal body fat stores with completion of the reproduction cycle. This allowance should be increased if lactation continues beyond this period or if maternal weight falls below the ideal weight for height. Obviously, allowances must be greater for women suckling more than one infant.

Table 12–4. SELENIUM CONCENTRATION OF HUMAN MILK

Area	City	N	Selenium (µg/liter)
High Se forage crops	Sioux Falls, S.D.	15	0.028
	Salt Lake City, Utah	14	0.022
	Billings, Mont.	10	0.021
Low Se forage crops	Syracuse, N.Y.	15	0.015
	Bristol, Conn.	15	0.015
	Akron, Ohio	15	0.013
Average 17 states		241	0.018

Table 12–5. RECOMMENDED DAILY DIETARY ALLOWANCE (1974) FOR FEMALES 19 TO 22 YEARS OF AGE

	Nonpregnant	Pregnant	Lactating
Energy (kcal)	2100	2400	2600
Protein (g)	46	76	66
Vitamin A (IU)	4000	5000	6000
Vitamin D (IU)	400	400	400
Vitamin E (IU)	12	15	15
Ascorbic acid (mg)	45	60	60
Folacin (μg)	400	800	600
Niacin (mg)	14	16	18
Riboflavin (mg)	1.4	1.7	1.9
Thiamine (mg)	1.1	1.4	1.4
Vitamin B_6 (mg)	2.0	2.5	2.5
Vitamin B_{12} (μg)	3.0	4.0	4.0
Calcium (mg)	800	1200	1200
Phosphorus (mg)	800	1200	1200
Iodine (μg)	100	125	150
Iron (mg)	18	18+	18
Magnesium (mg)	300	450	450
Zinc (mg)	15	20	25

English and Hitchcock compared the energy intake of 16 nursing women to 10 nonnursing women and found that the energy intake of breast-feeders in the sixth to eighth postpartum week was 2460 kcal (4). The energy intake of non-nursing mothers during this same postpartum period was 1880 kcal, a difference of 580 kcal. In a later study by Thomson and coworkers, lactating women were found to ingest 2716 kcal/day and nonnursing mothers 2125 kcal/day—a difference due to nursing of 591 kcal (30). By adding the assumed energy equivalents of body weight being lost, total energy available to the two groups was 2977 and 2364 kcal/day, respectively. If one assumes that the energy requirements for basal metabolism and activity are equivalent for the two groups, the energy for milk production can be calculated as 618 kcal. If the energy content of daily milk production is considered to be 560 kcal, the production efficiency for human milk is 90%.

The 20-g increment in RDA for protein for lactating women is recommended to cover the requirement for milk production with an allowance of 70% efficiency of protein utilization.

The increased energy and protein needs of lactation can be met by the mother's drinking somewhat less than an additional quart of milk per day. This will not provide, however, the increased recommendations for ascorbic acid, vitamin D, and folacin. The intake of other foods such as citrus fruits, vegetable oils, and meat must be slightly increased.

LACTATION AND DRUGS

Most drugs taken by the nursing mother will be excreted in her breast milk. The distribution of a compound across the membrane between plasma and milk is influenced by 1) its solubility in fat, 2) its degree of ionization, 3) its degree of protein binding, and 4) active versus passive transport including micro-phagocytosis.

Psychopharmacologic drugs such as chlorpromazine, codeine, heroin, morphine, Darvon, and dextroamphetamine do not appear to present problems for the nursing infant, although these drugs are secreted or excreted in breast milk (11, 20). Ethanol, but not its metabolite acetaldehyde, equilibrates rapidly between blood and breast milk following an acute loading dose (10). (Table 12–5). These observations have added significance in view of the effect of maternal alcohol ingestion during pregnancy on the fetus and newborn as described by Ouellette and Rosett (see Ch. 9, The Effect of Maternal Alcohol Ingestion During Pregnancy on Offspring).

LACTATION AND INFANT GROWTH

When the growth of formula-fed infants is compared to that of breast-fed infants, it is observed that most formula-fed infants have regained birth weight by the eighth day of life (8). Formula-fed infants continue to gain more rapidly in weight and length than breast-fed infants. These differences are considered to be energy related, reflecting differences in caloric intake rather than differences in composition of diet. Fomon attributes the greater gain in weight of formula-fed infants relative to breast-fed infants to overfeeding of the former (6). At the present time, the long-term consequences of such differences are a matter for speculation.

Several years ago we had an opportunity to study the effect of oral contraceptives on lactation. Milk production was evaluated in terms of infant weight gain. The average growth of breast-fed infants nursed by mothers not on oral contraceptives was 30 g/day. In contrast, infants nursed by mothers on oral contraceptives gained only 20 g/day. Similar results were reported by Miller and Hughes (17) and Koetsawang and coworkers (13). There was no question that oral contraceptives reduced milk production. Such observations pose a problem of considerable magnitude to a developing country like India, where family planning is desirable, yet the infant is solely dependent upon mother's milk for growth and development (2).

SPECULATION

The need to know more about factors that influence lactation in a quantitative as well as qualitative sense is no less acute now than it was 15 years ago. In the interim, while our scientific skills and understanding have increased, our society has become more complex. This combination can only mean more effort at understanding a very old process—lactation.

REFERENCES

1. Atkinson PJ, West RR: Loss of skeletal calcium in lactating women. J Obstet Gynaecol Br Commonw 77:555, 1970
2. Chopra JG: Effect of steroid contraceptives on lactation. Am J Clin Nutr 25:1202, 1972
3. Dirks OB, Jongeling–Eijndhoven JMPA, Flissebaalje TD, Gedalia I: Total and free ionic fluoride in human and cow's milk as determined by gas-liquid chromatography and the fluoride electrode. Caries Res 8:181, 1974
4. English RM, Hitchcock NE: Nutrient intakes during pregnancy, lactation and after the cessation of lactation in a group of Australian women. Br J Nutr 22:615, 1968
5. Filer LJ Jr, Mattson FH, Fomon SJ: Triglyceride configuration and fat absorption by the human infant. J Nutr 99:293, 1969
6. Fomon SJ: Infant Nutrition, 2nd ed. Philadelphia, WB Saunders, 1974, p 22
7. Fomon SJ: Infant Nutrition, 2nd ed. Philadelphia, WB Saunders, 1974, p 364
8. Fomon SJ, Thomas LN, Filer LJ Jr, Ziegler EE, Leonard MT: Food consumption and growth of normal infants fed milk-based formulas. Acta Paediat Scand [Suppl] 223:1–36, 1971
9. Insull W Jr, Hirsch J, James T, Ahrens EH: The fatty acids of human milk. II. Alterations produced by manipulation of caloric balance and exchange of dietary fats. J Clin Invest 38:443, 1959
10. Kesäniemi YA: Ethanol and acetaldehyde in the milk and peripheral blood of lactating women after ethanol administration. J Obstet Gynaecol Br Commonw 81:84, 1974
11. Knowles JA: Excretion of drugs in milk—a review. J Pediatr 80:401, 1972
12. Ko KW: Chemical composition of Korean human milk. J Korean Pediatr Assoc 9:13, 1966
13. Koetsawang S, Bhiraleus P, Chiemprajert T: Effects of oral contraceptives on lactation. Fertil Steril 23:24, 1972
14. Lindblad BS, Rahimtoola RJ: A pilot study of the quality of human milk in a lower socio-economic group in Karachi, Pakistan. Acta Paediatr Scand 63:125, 1974
15. Liu SH, Chu HI, Su CC, Yu TF, Cheng TY: Calcium and phosphorus metabolism in osteomalacia. IX. Metabolic behavior of infants fed on breast milk from mothers showing various states of vitamin D nutrition. J Clin Invest 19:327, 1940
16. Martinez GA: Personal communication
17. Miller GH, Hughes LR: Lactation and genital involution effects of a new low-dose oral contraceptive on breast-feeding mothers and their infants. Obstet Gynecol 35:44, 1970
18. NAS/NRC: Recommended Dietary Allowances, 8th ed., 1974
19. Newton M: Human lactation. In Kon SK, Cowie AT (eds): Milk: The Mammary Gland and Its Secretions, Vol I. New York, Academic Press, 1961, p 281
20. O'Brien TE: Excretion of drugs in human milk. Am J Hosp Pharm 31:844, 1974
21. PAG Bulletin: Breast feeding and weaning practices in developing countries and factors influencing them, Vol III, No. 4. Protein Advisory Group of the United Nations System, United Nations, New York, NY 10017, 1973
22. PAG Bulletin: Recommendations on policies and practices in infant and young child feeding and proposals for action to implement them, Vol V, No. 1. Protein Advisory Group of the United Nations System, United Nations, New York, NY 10017, 1975
23. Pitkin RM, Bahns JA, Filer LJ Jr, Reynolds WA: Mercury in human maternal and cord blood, placenta and milk. Proc Soc Exp Biol Med 151(3):565, 1976
24. Report on Employment and Earnings. Washington DC, Department of Labor Statistics, April, 1972
25. Shearer TR, Hadjimarkos DM: Geographic distribution of selenium in human milk. Arch Environ Health 30:230, 1975

26. Sinclair AJ, Crawford MA: The effect of a low-fat maternal diet on neonatal rats. Br
    J Nutr 29:127, 1973
27. Sjölin S: Den laga amningsfrekvensen i Sverige—vad gör vi? Stockholm, Semper IX
    Nutritions Symposium (Suppl No. 8), 1973
28. Sloper K, McKean L, Baum JD: Factors influencing breast feeding. Arch Dis Child
    50:165, 1975
29. Stegink LD, Filer LJ Jr, Baker GL: Monosodium glutamate: Effect on plasma and
    breast milk amino acid levels in lactating women. Proc Soc Exp Biol Med 140:836,
    1972
30. Thomson AM, Hytten FE, Billewicz WZ: The energy cost of human lactation. Br J
    Nutr 24:565, 1970

Chapter 13

Effect of Oral Contraceptives on Micronutrients and Changes in Trace Elements Due to Pregnancy

**Ananda S. Prasad, Kamran S. Moghissi, Kai Y. Lei,
Donald Oberleas, Joanne C. Stryker**

EFFECT OF ORAL CONTRACEPTIVES ON MICRONUTRIENTS

Estrogens and oral contraceptive agents (OCA) are widely used as prophylactic and therapeutic agents in gynecologic practice. It is estimated that 1 of 6 women of childbearing age in the United States currently uses OCA. These potent pharmacologic agents affect many aspects of human metabolism (8, 79). Alterations in the levels of iron, zinc, copper, calcium, and magnesium in the plasma as a result of OCA administration have been noted by many investigators (11, 12, 25, 60, 69, 73). Most of these studies, however, were performed in a small number of subjects and as such were limited in scope.

Various reviews in the literature indicate that use of OCA in women affects metabolism of vitamins (8, 79). Lumeng *et al.* (41) and Hontz *et al.* (22) observed a significant reduction of plasma pyridoxal phosphate (PLP) levels in OCA users. Our preliminary data (52) suggested that in the high income groups, plasma PLP levels were lower in OCA users as compared to those in controls. However, Brown *et al.* (9) found no differences in plasma PLP levels between OCA users and controls receiving controlled intakes of vitamin B_6. Larsson-Cohn (31) reported that serum glutamic oxaloacetic transaminase activities (SGOT) were abnormal in OCA users. Whereas SGOT is known to decrease as a result of vitamin B_6 deficiency (58), Aly *et al.* (3) showed that the activity of this enzyme in the red cell was higher in OCA users as compared to the controls.

Wertalik *et al.* (81) and Davis and Smith (17) observed a reduction in vitamin B_{12} levels in women taking OCA. The serum vitamin B_{12} binding capacity was also found to be increased in OCA users by Bianchine *et al.* (5). Reductions in serum folate levels in OCA users have been reported by Shojania *et al.* (70) and Streiff (76). Streiff also found that naturally occurring folate polyglutamates were poorly absorbed in volunteers taking OCA, although the monoglutamate was utilized normally. On the contrary, McLean *et al.* (44) and Pritchard *et al.* (57) found no alterations in the serum folate levels in OCA users. In addition, a slight increase in the average serum folic acid level in OCA users was reported by Castren and Rossi (13).

The purpose of this chapter is to document the effects of OCA on minerals and vitamins in a large number of subjects representing different socioeconomic groups.

METHODS

In prospective studies performed at Wayne State University, female subjects between the ages of 18 to 45 were divided into eight groups in a factorial arrangement with two socioeconomic levels and four different hormonal subgroups. The criteria of Myrianthopoulos and French (47) with an income adjustment were utilized in determining the division between the higher (A) and lower (B) socioeconomic classes. Subjects who were not taking OCA belonged to A-none or B-none groups. A-1 and B-1 groups consisted of those subjects who used Norinyl (1 mg norethindrone and 0.05 mg mestranol) for 3 months or more. A-2 and B-2 groups of subjects received Ovral (0.5 mg norgestrel and 0.005 mg of ethinyl estradiol) for 3 months or more. A-RP and B-RP groups consisted of women who resumed OCA within 5 weeks after pregnancy during lactation (Table 13–1).

Subjects were further divided in each group into supplemented and nonsupplemented subgroups according to whether or not they were taking vitamin and/or mineral supplementations.

Records of physical examinations by the physician and nutritional histories were recorded in each case on a form similar to those used in Interdepartment Committee on Nutrition for National Defense (ICNND) surveys (24). The number of subjects included in 24-hour recall dietary intake studies are shown in Table 13–2.

Hemoglobin, hematocrit, cell indices, and peripheral blood smears were examined according to routine methods (83). Plasma total protein and serum iron were determined by Technicon AutoAnalyzer methods (78). The cellulose acetate electrophoresis technique (86) was used for plasma protein fractionation. Plasma copper, zinc, magnesium, and calcium levels were assayed by atomic absorption spectrophotometry (54). Erythrocyte zinc and magnesium were also determined (54).

Plasma vitamin A and carotene levels were determined by the modified Carr–Price method (24) and plasma vitamin C levels were assayed by a modified method of Roe and Kenther (24). Grab samples of urine were collected from subjects for thiamine and riboflavin determinations. Urinary levels of thiamine and riboflavin were measured fluorometrically by modified methods of Consolazio *et al.* (24) and Slater and Morell (24), respectively. Creatinine levels in the urine were determined on a Technicon AutoAnalyzer using a modified procedure of Folin and Wu (78).

Plasma pyridoxal phosphate was determined by simple enzymatic assay (14). Erythrocyte glutamic oxalacetic transaminase (EGOT) was measured in a hemolysate of red blood cells (59). The cells were washed with 0.85% sodium chloride

Table 13–1. NUMBER OF SUBJECTS IN THE CLINICAL AND BIOCHEMICAL STUDIES

OCA use	Socioeconomic group	
	A	B
None	128	98
Pill 1	35	111
Pill 2	44	124
Resume pill (RP)	78	105

OCA, oral contraceptive agent.

Table 13–2. NUMBER OF SUBJECTS IN THE 24-HOUR DIETARY RECALL STUDY

OCA use	Socioeconomic group	
	A	B
None	49	49
Pill 1	30	46
Pill 2	25	49
Resume pill (RP)	42	47

OCA, oral contraceptive agent.

Table 13–3. TREATMENT COMPARISONS IN ANALYSIS OF VARIANCE

Treatment	Degree of freedom
P_1 = None vs. Norinyl, Ovral, and RP	1
P_2 = RP vs. Norinyl and Ovral	1
P_3 = Norinyl vs. Ovral	1
I = Income	1
S = Supplement	1
Interactions	10
$I \times P_1$	1
$I \times P_2$	1
$I \times P_3$	1
$S \times P_1$	1
$S \times P_2$	1
$S \times P_3$	1
$I \times S$	1
$I \times S \times P_1$	1
$I \times S \times P_2$	1
$I \times S \times P_3$	1

solution and diluted with saline in the proportion of 0.8 ml saline to 1 ml packed cells. The test was carried out on 0.1 ml of a 1:20 hemolysate. For measurement of PLP stimulation, 0.1 ml hemolysate was incubated with 0.1 ml of PLP (0.5 mg/ml) for 20 minutes at 37°C prior to the colorimetric determination of EGOT.

Erythrocyte and plasma folic acid were determined by a microbiologic assay using *Lactobacillus casei* (34). Serum vitamin B_{12} levels were measured by a microbiologic assay using *Lactobacillus leichmannii* (74).

Nutritional and biochemical data were analyzed statistically by analysis of variance (Table 13–3). Missing data were processed by the procedure of least squares analysis of variance (82). Means were ranked by the Duncan's New Multiple Range Test (82). Clinical data were statistically analyzed by chi-square (82).

RESULTS

The incidence of dry skin, easily pluckable hair, angular lesions of the mouth, caries and debris of teeth, marginal redness, swelling and bleeding of the gums, filiform papillary atrophy, fungiform papillary hypertrophy of the tongue and glossitis, and scaling of skin were more frequently observed in the B groups than in the A groups. In the A groups, some of the above clinical signs were most common in the nonsupplemented groups of subjects. These data have been

Table 13–4. INCIDENCE OF CLINICAL ABNORMALITIES (PERCENT OF ABNORMALITIES)

	Socio economic group	None	Pill 1	Pill 2	RP	P values None vs pill 1	None vs pill 2	None vs RP
Hair								
Dry-brittle	A	15.0	24.3	18.2	5.2	—	—	0.03
	B	33.0	36.3	16.3	30.5	—	0.005	—
Easily pluckable	A	9.4	18.9	13.6	3.1	—	—	—
	B	22.3	36.6	12.2	24.8	0.03	—	—
Lips								
Angular lesions	A	1.6	10.8	15.9	2.1	0.02	0.001	—
	B	14.5	17.9	8.9	23.8	—	—	0.05
Teeth								
Caries (4+)	A	7.9	45.9	40.9	7.2	0.001	0.001	—
	B	48.5	54.5	41.5	51.4	—	—	—
Debris or calculus	A	8.7	35.1	31.8	7.2	0.003	0.001	—
	B	48.0	54.5	27.6	44.7	0.03	—	—
Tongue								
Filiform papillary atrophy	A	1.6	0.0	2.3	1.0	—	—	—
	B	7.8	6.3	5.7	8.6	—	—	—
Fungiform papillary hypertrophy	A	0	0	2.3	0	—	—	—
	B	1.9	1.8	2.4	4.8	—	—	—
Gums								
Marginal redness	L	5.5	35.1	31.8	4.1			
or swelling	A D	0.0	2.7	2.3	1.0	0.001	0.001	—
	L	33.0	29.5	27.6	26.7			
	B D	5.8	15.2	8.1	14.3	—	—	—
Swollen red	A L	2.4	16.2	22.7	3.1			
papillae	D	0.0	8.1	6.8	1.0	0.001	0.001	—
	B L	17.8	30.4	22.0	20.0			
	D	5.8	5.4	8.1	6.7	—	—	—
Bleeding gums	A L	4.7	18.9	6.8	1.0			
	D	0.0	2.7	6.8	0.0	0.003	0.01	—
	B L	10.7	15.2	17.1	8.6			
	D	4.9	4.5	6.5	4.8	—	—	—
Skin								
Dry	A	2.4	10.8	9.1	3.1	—	—	—
scaling	B	12.6	19.6	8.1	19.0	—	—	—
(xerosis)								

L, localized; D, diffused.

Table 13-5. INTAKE OF CALORIES, PROTEIN, CALCIUM, MAGNESIUM, IRON, COPPER, AND ZINC IN SUPPLEMENTED AND NONSUPPLEMENTED SUBJECTS TAKING ORAL CONTRACEPTIVE AGENTS (MEAN ± SD)

	Kilocalories			Protein (g)			Calcium (mg)			Magnesium (mg)		
	S	NS	Av	S	NS	Av	S	NS	Av	S	NS	Av
A-None	1275 ±520	1448 ±378	1342 ±473	62.8 ±25.6	69.8 ±17.6	65.5 ±22.9	606 ±456	563 ±288	589 ±397	155 ±78	139 ±50	149 ±69
A-1	1539 ±761	1400 ±640	1436 ±670	68.1 ±343	71.8 ±26.7	70.9 ±28.3	551 ±408	432 ±246	460 ±288	179 ±168	140 ±64	149 ±96
A-2	1543 ±415	1575 ±723	1569 ±665	89.9 ±32.0	84.2 ±40.9	85.3 ±38.7	475 ±473	450 ±328	463 ±350	189 ±82	169 ±77	173 ±77
A-RP	2432 ±785	1364 ±446	2152 ±852	111.2 ±37.3	74.4 ±35.5	101.5 ±39.9	1200 ±575	431 ±324	998 ±620	280 ±116	162 ±95	249 ±121
B-none	1394 ±448	1650 ±903	1582 ±811	64.4 ±23.7	68.4 ±31.5	67.4 ±29.5	568 ±340	424 ±327	462 ±333	143 ±46	150 ±74	148 ±68
B-1	1491 ±313	1474 ±574	1476 ±540	70.2 ±23.3	72.1 ±30.1	71.8 ±29.0	360 ±179	456 ±339	442 ±320	154 ±34	154 ±72	154 ±67
B-2	1433 ±728	1341 ±503	1360 ±548	72.7 ±46.9	61.0 ±24.9	63.4 ±30.4	375 ±273	402 ±297	396 ±290	125 ±48	144 ±74	140 ±70
B-RP	1596 ±683	1436 ±675	1494 ±675	69.5 ±27.8	58.6 ±33.8	62.5 ±31.9	456 ±299	365 ±285	398 ±290	153 ±68	122 ±59	133 ±64
P values*	P_1 0.06 P_2 0.001 IP_1 0.015			P_1 0.01 IP_1 0.02 I 0.001			P_2 0.001 IP_2 0.001 I 0.001 S 0.001			P_1 0.02 P_2 0.02 IP_1 0.03 IP_2 0.01 S 0.01 IS 0.03		

S, supplemented; NS, nonsupplemented; Av, average
*See Table 13–3 for abbreviations.

Table 13-5. INTAKE OF CALORIES, PROTEIN, CALCIUM, MAGNESIUM, IRON, COPPER, AND ZINC IN SUPPLEMENTED AND NONSUPPLEMENTED SUBJECTS TAKING ORAL CONTRACEPTIVE AGENTS (MEAN ± SD) (continued)

	Iron (mg)			Copper (mg)			Zinc (mg)		
	S	NS	Av	S	NS	Av	S	NS	Av
A-None	16.7 ±8.7	12.0 ±5.6	14.8 ±7.9	1.66 ±0.90	1.31 ±0.52	1.52 ±0.79	9.60 ±5.62	11.84 ±6.92	10.5 ±9.6
A-1	21.4 ±6.8	9.0 ±4.4	11.9 ±7.2	1.33 ±0.73	1.43 ±0.78	1.40 ±0.76	9.97 ±9.80	12.34 ±7.68	12.1 ±8.0
A-2	27.1 ±3.2	10.7 ±6.9	14.0 ±9.2	1.27 ±0.51	1.58 ±0.97	1.52 ±0.90	10.30 ±7.87	11.50 ±6.80	11.3 ±6.9
A-RP	97.6 ±78.6	9.5 ±3.8	74.6 ±77.9	3.09 ±1.38	1.49 ±0.79	2.67 ±1.44	17.65 ±8.05	11.06 ±12.37	15.9 ±9.7
B-none	39.3 ±39.5	10.0 ±5.1	17.8 ±24.1	1.38 ±0.66	1.37 ±0.79	1.37 ±0.65	10.51 ±7.95	10.50 ±6.66	10.5 ±6.9
B-1	31.6 ±34.2	9.6 ±4.0	13.0 ±15.3	1.01 ±0.39	1.41 ±0.87	1.35 ±0.82	9.91 ±4.19	8.33 ±5.91	8.6 ±5.7
B-2	36.2 ±38.9	8.3 ±3.6	13.9 ±20.6	1.22 ±0.52	1.28 ±0.69	1.27 ±0.65	13.98 ±10.95	9.44 ±8.74	10.4 ±9.3
B-RP	22.1 ±14.5	8.4 ±4.1	13.3 ±11.3	1.22 ±0.66	1.13 ±0.58	1.16 ±0.60	12.24 ±11.10	9.69 ±8.22	10.6 ±9.3

P values*

Iron (mg): P_1 0.001, P_2 0.001, IP_1 0.001, IP_2 0.001, I 0.005, S 0.001

Copper (mg): P_1 0.07, P_2 0.001, IP_1 0.02, IP_2 0.001, I 0.001, S 0.01, IS 0.01

Zinc (mg): P_2 0.05, I 0.03

S, supplementd; NS, nonsupplemented; Av, average
*See Table 13–3 for abbreviations.

Table 13–6. INTAKE OF VITAMINS A AND C, THIAMINE, RIBOFLAVIN, FOLIC ACID, AND VITAMIN B_6 IN SUPPLEMENTED AND NONSUPPLEMENTED SUBJECTS TAKING ORAL CONTRACEPTIVE AGENTS (MEAN±SD)

	Vitamin A (IU)			Vitamin C (mg)			Thiamine (mg)		
	S	NS	Av	S	NS	Av	S	NS	Av
A-none	11307 ±8546	3229 ±2568	8175 ±7900	203 ±233	58 ±50	147 ±191	5.50 ±6.13	0.99 ±0.68	3.75 ±5.28
A-1	6256 ±3766	3340 ±3396	4020 ±3641	223 ±223	58 ±64	96 ±197	2.22 ±2.44	0.95 ±0.82	1.25 ±1.43
A-2	7915 ±9167	3971 ±4458	4680 ±5698	96 ±83	65 ±72	71 ±74	1.80 ±1.29	0.73 ±0.45	0.95 ±0.79
A-RP	12581 ±11496	3806 ±3941	10283 ±10758	191 ±155	81 ±67	162 ±145	4.41 ±2.49	1.02 ±0.71	3.53 ±2.63
B-none	6456 ±4540	3646 ±4170	4392 ±4405	46 ±28	59 ±61	63 ±75	3.06 ±2.13	0.96 ±0.55	1.52 ±1.49
B-1	5717 ±4694	6641 ±12236	6500 ±11380	123 ±104	54 ±81	65 ±87	2.73 ±1.92	1.18 ±0.86	1.41 ±1.20
B-2	6473 ±4307	3637 ±6205	4215 ±5941	130 ±150	59 ±71	74 ±96	3.06 ±2.11	1.14 ±0.86	1.53 ±1.44
B-RP	8168 ±6373	3339 ±3861	5086 ±5388	76 ±60	46 ±40	57 ±50	2.40 ±1.49	1.09 ±0.64	1.56 ±1.20
P values*	S 0.001 IS 0.04			I 0.001 S 0.001 IS 0.01			P, 0.05 S 0.001		

S, supplemented; NS, nonsupplemented; Av, average.
*See Table 13–3 for abbreviations.

Table 13-6. INTAKE OF VITAMINS A AND C, THIAMINE, RIBOFLAVIN, FOLIC ACID, AND VITAMIN B_6 IN SUPPLEMENTED AND NONSUPPLEMENTED SUBJECTS TAKING ORAL CONTRACEPTIVE AGENTS (MEAN±SD) (continued)

	Riboflavin (mg)			Folic acid (µg)			Vitamin B_6 (mg)		
	S	NS	Av	S	NS	Av	S	NS	Av
A-none	5.23 ±4.77	1.30 ±0.54	3.70 ±4.20	94.3 ±61.5	73.1 ±52.5	86.1 ±58.6	3.24 ±2.38	1.19 ±0.57	2.45 ±2.14
A-1	2.58 ±1.74	1.10 ±0.50	1.45 ±1.10	120.0 ±113.6	79.2 ±63.4	92.6 ±78.8	2.04 ±1.66	1.31 ±0.65	1.55 ±1.01
A-2	1.91 ±1.34	1.32 ±0.88	1.43 ±0.99	103.4 ±37.3	63.5 ±58.2	71.5 ±56.3	1.93 ±0.92	0.98 ±0.63	1.17 ±0.78
A-RP	4.46 ±1.91	1.25 ±0.56	3.62 ±2.19	430.9 ±412.4	94.3 ±78.4	342.7 ±385.2	5.70 ±6.04	1.17 ±0.58	4.51 ±5.55
B-none	2.95 ±1.90	1.13 ±0.56	1.62 ±1.34	81.5 ±58.7	89.3 ±70.5	87.3 ±67.1	1.72 ±0.67	1.02 ±0.54	1.21 ±0.65
B-1	2.72 ±1.82	1.34 ±1.26	1.55 ±1.43	77.3 ±49.1	117.5 ±94.7	111.4 ±90.0	1.98 ±0.99	0.88 ±0.47	1.05 ±0.69
B-2	2.99 ±1.91	1.18 ±0.71	1.55 ±1.27	76.2 ±52.3	81.0 ±72.5	80.0 ±68.4	1.62 ±0.86	0.97 ±0.59	1.10 ±0.69
B-RP	2.76 ±1.63	1.09 ±0.65	1.69 ±1.36	109.3 ±89.6	72.8 ±80.8	86.0 ±84.9	1.73 ±0.98	1.05 ±0.57	1.29 ±0.80
P values*		P_1 0.05 I 0.01 S 0.001 IS 0.05			P_1 0.001 P_2 0.001 IP_1 0.05 IP_2 0.001 I 0.005 S 0.001 IS 0.001			P_2 0.001 IP_2 0.002 I 0.001 S 0.001 IS 0.005	

S, supplemented; NS, nonsupplemented; Av, average.
*See Table 13–3 for abbreviations.

Table 13–7. LEVELS OF HEMOGLOBIN, HEMATOCRIT, RED BLOOD CELL COUNT, SERUM IRON, AND TOTAL IRON-BINDING CAPACITY IN SUPPLEMENTED AND NONSUPPLEMENTED SUBJECTS TAKING ORAL CONTRACEPTIVE AGENTS (MEAN ± SD)

	Hemoglobin (gm/100 ml)			Hematocrit (%)			Red blood cell count ($10^6 \times mm^3$)		
	S	NS	Av	S	NS	Av	S	NS	Av
A-none	13.66 ±1.86	13.14 ±1.48	13.45 ±1.73	41.01 ±4.27	40.54 ±3.03	40.82 ±3.80	4.644 ±1.163	4.632 +0.690	4.640 +1.001
A-1	13.66 ±1.52	13.09 ±1.47	13.22 ±1.48	40.38 ±3.66	41.33 ±4.06	41.11 ±3.94	4.389 ±0.652	4.676 ±1.132	4.591 ±1.010
A-2	13.30 ±2.22	13.05 ±1.13	13.10 ±1.40	41.00 ±4.80	41.47 ±3.72	41.37 ±3.92	4.656 ±1.125	4.590 ±0.891	4.603 ±0.927
A-RP	12.01 ±1.39	12.39 ±1.85	12.08 ±1.48	36.27 ±4.00	38.67 ±5.47	36.73 ±4.39	4.125 ±0.834	4.347 ±0.781	4.161 ±0.825
B-none	13.30 ±1.50	12.80 ±1.68	12.93 ±1.64	40.20 ±3.35	39.56 ±4.25	39.72 ±4.04	4.984 ±1.594	4.534 ±0.867	4.636 ±1.079
B-1	12.67 ±1.86	12.97 ±1.84	12.92 ±1.84	38.64 ±4.77	40.73 ±4.35	40.40 ±4.46	5.480 ±1.833	5.595 ±1.340	5.572 ±1.433
B-2	12.98 ±1.35	13.49 ±1.47	13.40 ±1.46	40.09 ±3.44	40.65 ±5.32	40.55 ±5.03	4.659 ±0.637	4.804 ±1.001	4.778 ±0.945
B-RP	13.38 ±1.69	13.15 ±1.70	13.23 ±1.69	40.86 ±3.87	40.27 ±3.72	40.47 ±3.76	4.704 ±0.816	4.800 ±0.967	4.764 ±0.914
P values*	P_2 0.05 IP_2 0.05	P_2 0.05 IP_2 0.05			P_2 0.05 IP_2 0.05			I 0.05	

S, supplemented; NS, nonsupplemented; Av, average.
*See Table 13–3 for abbreviations.

Table 13–7. LEVELS OF HEMOGLOBIN, HEMATOCRIT, RED BLOOD CELL COUNT, SERUM IRON, AND TOTAL IRON-BUILDING CAPACITY IN SUPPLEMENTED AND NONSUPPLEMENTED SUBJECTS TAKING ORAL CONTRACEPTIVE AGENTS (MEAN ± SD) (continued)

	Serum iron (ug/100 ml)			Serum total iron-binding capacity (µg/100 ml)		
	S	NS	Av	S	NS	Av
A-none	95.89 ±35.99	81.16 ±24.84	89.68 ±32.49	267.1 ±81.0	271.0 ±68.1	268.7 ±75.7
A-1	89.00 ±30.75	100.93 ±37.16	98.20 ±35.73	318.4 ±81.7	311.5 ±65.8	312.9 ±68.0
A-2	84.80 ±34.88	87.42 ±39.86	86.81 ±38.38	317.6 ±59.8	345.4 ±92.1	338.9 ±85.9
A-RP	50.40 ±29.97	47.75 ±24.99	49.89 ±28.95	305.2 ±65.7	307.0 ±76.9	305.6 ±67.5
B-none	69.04 ±34.43	69.68 ±34.43	69.38 ±34.43	292.5 ±67.6	312.1 ±86.2	307.3 ±82.6
B-1	99.52 ±19.71	90.07 ±28.84	91.53 ±27.77	305.6 ±70.2	337.4 ±72.5	332.5 ±72.7
B-2	74.14 ±30.94	75.53 ±30.02	75.27 ±30.06	305.1 ±57.8	335.4 ±80.6	330.0 ±77.6
B-RP	73.15 ±39.51	69.40 ±37.73	70.71 ±38.20	304.4 ±111.9	316.0 ±91.6	311.8 ±99.1
P values*	P_1 0.03 P_2 0.001 IP_1 0.001				P_1 0.001 IP_1 0.02 I 0.06 S 0.02	

S, supplemented; NS, nonsupplemented; Av, average.
*See Table 13–3 for abbreviations.

reported in detail elsewhere (55). In the A groups, higher incidences of angular lesions of the mouth, caries and debris of the teeth, and marginal redness, swelling, and bleeding of the gums were seen in the OCA users than in the controls (Table 13–4). The incidences of easily pluckable hair, angular lesions of the mouth, and debris or calculus of the teeth were more frequently observed in the B-1 group as compared to the B-none group. Higher incidence of angular lesions of the mouth was seen in the B-RP group as compared to the B-none group.

Table 13–5 shows the intake of calories, protein, calcium, magnesium, iron, copper, and zinc in the subjects. In general, the intake of calories, protein, calcium, magnesium, iron, copper, and zinc in subjects using OCA did not differ from the controls. Group A subjects' consumption of protein, calcium, magnesium, iron, copper, and zinc was found to be higher than that of group B subjects. The caloric, protein, calcium, magnesium, iron, copper, and zinc intakes of the A-RP group were higher than those of the A-none, A-1, and A-2 groups. As expected, the supplemented group consumed greater amounts of calcium, iron, magnesium, and copper. However, for magnesium and copper, this supplementation effect was seen only in the A groups.

In general, the OCA subjects' intake of vitamin A, C, B_6 and folic acid did not differ from the controls. However, the intake of thiamine and riboflavin in A-1 and A-2 appeared to be lower than the A-none subjects. The A-RP group of subjects had higher intake of vitamin B_6 and folic acid than A-1 and A-2 subjects. As expected, the subjects from the supplemented groups had higher intake of vitamin A, C, B_6, thiamine, riboflavin, and folic acid than the nonsupplemented groups, and the A groups had higher intake of vitamin C, B_6, riboflavin, and folic acid than the B groups. Dietary intake of vitamin A, C, B_6, folic acid, and riboflavin of the supplemented groups was higher than the nonsupplemented groups in A but not in B (Table 13–6).

Table 13–7 shows the changes in hemoglobin, hematocrit, red blood cell (RBC) count, serum iron, and iron-binding capacity in different groups of subjects. No effect of OCA use was seen on hemoglobin, hematocrit, or RBC count. Whereas serum iron was increased in both A and B groups due to Norinyl, there was no effect due to Ovral. Total iron-binding capacity (TIBC) was increased as a result of OCA administration in A and B groups. In group A-RP, a decrease in hemoglobin, hematocrit, RBC count, and serum iron was observed; TIBC was increased in both A-RP and B-RP groups. In general, the TIBC values were higher in the B groups as compared to the A groups and in the nonsupplemented groups as compared to the supplemented groups.

Table 13–8 shows the results of copper and zinc analysis. Plasma copper was increased in A and B groups as a result of OCA administration. No effect on plasma copper levels due to socioeconomic status was observed. Plasma copper was also increased in both A-RP and B-RP groups. Plasma zinc decreased as a result of OCA administration in A and B groups. An increase in the RBC zinc was observed due to administration of Norinyl in both A and B groups. A decrease in plasma zinc and an increase in RBC zinc levels was observed in the

A-RP group only. Although no socioeconomic effect was observed in plasma zinc levels, A groups showed higher RBC zinc concentrations as compared to B groups. With respect to plasma calcium and magnesium and RBC magnesium concentrations, no significant effect of OCA administration was observed.

Table 13–9 shows the results of plasma total protein and serum albumin determination in different groups. Although there was no effect of OCA administration on plasma total protein, the levels of serum albumin were decreased due to intake of OCA in both groups. Serum albumin levels were significantly lower in A-RP as compared to A-none, A-1, and A-2 groups.

Plasma vitamin A levels were increased due to OCA administration in both A and B groups of subjects (Table 13–10). Supplemented subjects had higher levels of plasma vitamin A. No socioeconomic effect was observed. Plasma carotene levels were decreased due to OCA administration, and group A subjects had higher levels of plasma carotene. Plasma ascorbate was not affected by OCA administration. Group A subjects had higher plasma ascorbate levels as compared to group B. Supplemented subjects had higher plasma ascorbate levels as compared to nonsupplemented subjects.

Table 13–11 shows the results of urinary excretion of thiamine and riboflavin in various groups of subjects. Urinary excretion of both vitamins was decreased in subjects using OCA in A and A-RP groups. Group A subjects had higher excretion of thiamine and riboflavin as compared to group B subjects. Effects of supplementation were observed in group A only.

Results of PLP, EGOT, and percent stimulation of EGOT are presented in Table 13–12. In group A, the plasma PLP level was decreased due to OCA administration. Supplementation effect was seen mainly in the A groups. Plasma PLP was found to be lower in the A-RP group than in the A-1 and A-2 groups.

EGOT activities were found to be lower in the RP and OCA groups. This reduction in activities due to OCA was greater in the B groups as compared to A groups. Supplementation effect was seen in both groups. The percent stimulation of EGOT was found to be greater in the OCA and RP groups. No socioeconomic or supplementation effect was seen so far as the EGOT stimulation test was concerned.

Table 13–13 shows the results of erythrocyte and serum folate and vitamin B_{12} determinations. Both plasma and red cell folate levels were higher in group A than in group B. Supplementation effect was seen in both groups. Erythrocyte and serum folate in the RP groups were higher than in the OCA groups.

The Duncan's New Multiple Range Test indicated that the A-RP subjects had higher red cell and serum folate concentrations than A-none subjects (Table 13–14). Erythrocyte folate in A-1 and A-2 groups was decreased in comparison to subjects in A-none and A-RP groups. The level of serum folate in A-2 group only was decreased when compared to A-none and A-RP groups.

Serum vitamin B_{12} levels in A-1 and B-1 groups were lower than A-2 and B-2 groups. No other significant differences were found with respect to serum vitamin B_{12} levels.

Table 13–8. PLASMA COPPER AND ZINC, AND ERYTHROCYTE ZINC LEVELS IN SUPPLEMENTED AND NONSUPPLEMENTED SUBJECTS TAKING ORAL CONTRACEPTIVE AGENTS (MEAN ±SD)

	Plasma copper (µg/100 ml)			Plasma zinc (µg/100 ml)			Erythrocyte zinc (µg/gm hemoglobin)		
	S	NS	Av	S	NS	Av	S	NS	Av
A-none	138.8 ±102.3	126.8 ±38.0	133.8 ±82.3	117.35 ±21.98	119.04 ±16.08	118.04 ±19.74	39.26 ±5.87	40.05 ±7.89	39.58 ±6.73
A-1	230.5 ±73.0	244.9 ±51.1	241.6 ±55.9	109.00 ±21.67	112.89 ±15.97	112.00 ±17.16	36.14 ±7.89	43.08 ±10.05	41.28 ±9.89
A-2	221.6 ±52.9	227.8 ±49.1	226.3 ±49.4	120.40 ±16.05	114.06 ±17.32	115.54 ±17.07	40.84 ±7.22	38.86 ±6.73	39.25 ±6.76
A-RP	245.0 ±63.3	209.3 ±54.9	238.9 ±63.2	108.08 ±21.95	102.53 ±12.25	107.01 ±20.49	45.21 ±10.83	47.98 ±12.64	45.66 ±11.10
B-none	143.8 ±35.0	141.7 ±33.6	142.2 ±33.8	117.68 ±20.89	119.36 ±26.40	118.93 ±25.02	37.71 ±10.95	36.61 ±7.11	36.85 ±7.94
B-1	251.5 ±93.8	222.8 ±57.8	227.5 ±65.2	111.77 ±12.45	113.27 ±16.95	113.04 ±16.29	42.53 ±12.49	41.05 ±7.26	41.34 ±8.38
B-2	211.7 ±232.1	232.1 ±86.2	228.5 ±80.6	112.43 ±22.72	116.56 ±24.81	115.83 ±24.42	37.00 ±6.87	36.97 ±6.89	36.98 ±6.85
B-RP	217.8 ±64.1	231.2 ±63.4	226.4 ±63.6	115.22 ±19.78	115.28 ±40.41	115.26 ±34.38	42.48 ±6.93	41.55 ±9.63	41.86 ±8.78
P values*	P_1 0.001				P_1 0.003			P_1 0.001 P_2 0.001 I 0.01 S 0.01 IS 0.002	

S, supplemented; NS, nonsupplemented; Av average.
*See Table 13–3 for abbreviations.

Table 13–9. LEVELS OF PLASMA TOTAL PROTEIN AND SERUM ALBUMIN IN SUPPLEMENTED AND NONSUPPLEMENTED SUBJECTS TAKING ORAL CONTRACEPTIVE AGENTS (MEAN ±SD)

	Plasma total protein (g/100 ml)			Serum albumin (g/100 ml)		
	S	NS	Av	S	NS	Av
A-none	7.216 ±0.592	7.358 ±0.662	7.275 ±0.623	4.045 ±0.612	4.008 ±0.507	4.03 ±0.57
A-1	7.650 ±0.351	7.659 ±0.445	7.657 ±0.420	3.892 ±0.494	3.714 ±0.520	3.75 ±0.51
A-2	7.660 ±0.924	7.624 ±0.726	7.633 ±0.765	3.638 ±0.620	3.731 ±0.557	3.71 ±0.57
A-RP	6.835 ±0.705	7.153 ±0.839	6.900 ±0.738	3.323 ±0.402	3.413 ±0.516	3.34 ±0.42
B-none	7.737 ±0.642	7.588 ±1.204	7.624 ±1.082	3.907 ±0.553	3.879 ±0.817	3.89 ±0.75
B-1	7.712 ±0.499	7.464 ±0.839	7.502 ±0.799	3.605 ±0.711	3.502 ±0.661	3.52 ±0.67
B-2	7.355 ±1.036	7.785 ±0.538	7.707 ±0.672	3.665 ±0.642	3.867 ±0.532	3.83 ±0.55
B-RP	7.473 ±0.687	7.483 ±0.633	7.480 ±0.649	3.718 ±0.535	3.666 ±0.435	3.68 ±0.47
P values*		P_2 0.001 IP_2 0.005 I 0.001			P_1 0.001 P_2 0.01 P_3 0.001 IP_1 0.02 IP_2 0.005 IP_3 0.03 IP_3 0.03	

S, supplemented; NS, nonsupplemented; Av, average.
*See Table 13–3 for abbreviations.

Table 13–10. LEVELS OF PLASMA VITAMIN A AND CAROTENE AND ASCORBIC ACID IN SUPPLEMENTED AND NONSUPPLEMENTED USERS OF ORAL CONTRA-
CEPTIVE AGENTS (MEAN ± SD)

	Vitamin A (μg/100 ml)			Carotene (μg/100 ml)			Ascorbic Acid (mg/100 ml)		
	S	NS	Av	S	NS	Av	S	NS	Av
A-none	50.94 ±15.75	50.01 ±13.54	50.57 ±14.85	88.87 ±29.99	78.32 ±32.46	84.51 ±31.35	1.34 ±0.57	0.90 ±0.37	1.15 ±0.54
A-1	67.56 ±26.09	60.55 ±24.19	62.15 ±24.42	55.33 ±14.82	69.03 ±19.33	65.90 ±19.11	0.89 ±0.63	0.73 ±0.35	0.77 ±0.43
A-2	67.25 ±19.19	61.57 ±17.31	62.86 ±17.68	61.68 ±20.52	60.97 ±22.34	61.13 ±21.71	1.01 ±0.46	0.76 ±0.37	0.82 ±0.40
A-RP	59.92 ±21.74	64.78 ±15.81	60.86 ±20.73	88.07 ±94.89	60.76 ±23.30	82.82 ±86.41	1.11 ±0.56	0.93 ±0.43	1.08 ±0.54
B-none	52.43 ±17.55	43.32 ±17.57	45.51 ±17.56	61.45 ±24.24	65.63 ±56.34	64.50 ±50.32	0.64 ±0.30	0.75 ±0.45	0.71 ±0.39
B-1	55.18 ±17.91	56.62 ±15.72	56.40 ±16.00	53.01 ±11.74	63.99 ±20.17	62.31 ±19.49	0.78 ±0.42	0.73 ±0.40	0.74 ±0.40
B-2	63.55 ±21.57	56.84 ±19.73	58.06 ±20.15	51.06 ±17.31	57.54 ±18.91	56.35 ±18.73	0.73 ±0.38	0.69 ±0.37	0.70 ±0.37
B-RP	66.19 ±16.84	60.44 ±19.10	62.53 ±18.43	53.00 ±18.89	56.56 ±18.06	55.28 ±18.35	0.72 ±0.44	0.69 ±0.35	0.70 ±0.39
P values*	P_1 0.001 S 0.06			P_1 0.01 I 0.001			I 0.001 S 0.001 IS 0.001		

S, supplemented; NS, nonsupplemented; Ave, average.
*See Table 13–3 for abbreviations.

175

Table 13–11. URINARY LEVELS OF THIAMINE AND RIBOFLAVIN IN SUPPLEMENTED AND NONSUPPLEMENTED ORAL CONTRACEPTIVE USERS (MEAN ± SD)

	Urinary thiamine (µg/g creatinine)			Urinary riboflavin (µg/g creatinine)		
	S	NS	Av	S	NS	Av
A-none	884.9 ±1088.6	363.2 ±451.7	671.1 ±918.9	1200.6 ±1393.3	343.8 ±529.1	853.6 ±1199.6
A-1	488.5 ±211.3	302.8 ±215.4	346.6 ±225.8	333.0 ±263.0	322.6 ±324.6	324.9 ±307.9
A-2	387.7 ±597.2	246.8 ±184.8	275.6 ±310.9	563.6 ±740.0	318.8 ±320.4	368.8 ±439.2
A-RP	533.6 ±990.2	251.9 ±110.1	480.3 ±898.3	680.9 ±1185.8	318.5 ±350.6	608.4 ±1079.7
B-none	372.0 ±370.0	282.6 ±372.7	306.6 ±372.0	589.3 ±110.4	239.1 ±244.9	333.0 ±621.1
B-1	252.8 ±147.1	325.5 ±492.0	314.2 ±456.1	291.5 ±177.4	429.7 ±765.2	408.7 ±709.1
B-2	267.7 ±238.3	256.2 ±210.4	258.2 ±214.4	239.2 ±219.8	238.6 ±227.6	238.7 ±225.4
B-RP	279.8 ±263.4	301.6 ±411.0	293.9 ±285.8	252.7 ±284.8	314.4 ±762.1	292.4 ±633.2
P values*		P_1 0.005 IP_1 0.08 I 0.003 S 0.001 IS 0.003			P_1 0.01 I 0.001 S 0.001 IS 0.01	

S, supplemented; NS, nonsupplemented; Av, average.
*See Table 13–3 for abbreviations.

Table 13–12. LEVELS OF PLASMA PYRIDOXAL PHOSPHATE, ERYTHROCYTE GLUTAMIC OXALACETIC TRANSAMINASE, AND PERCENT STIMULATION OF EGOT (MEAN ± SD)

	Plasma PLP (ng/ml)			EGOT RF Units*			Percent stimulation of EGOT		
	S	NS	Av	S	NS	Av	S	NS	Av
A-none	27.3 ±15.2	12.6 ±7.3	18.5 ±13.1 (25)	4.01 ±1.86	2.83 ±1.02	3.61 ±1.71 (82)	132 ±76	163 ±91	143 ±82 (81)
A-1	9.5 ±5.7	10.6 ±4.6	10.3 ±4.9 (14)	2.43 ±1.97	3.70 ±2.57	3.41 ±2.43 (13)	252 ±115	188 ±174	203 ±160 (13)
A-2	11.7 ±8.6	7.8 ±2.8	9.0 ±6.3 (16)	3.37 ±0.06	3.21 ±1.61	3.25 ±1.40 (13)	162 ±40	166 ±136	165 ±119 (13)
A-RP	6.2 ±5.1	6.6 ±3.0	6.3 ±4.8 (65)	3.87 ±2.16	3.35 ±1.81	3.57 ±1.81 (7)	117 ±33	200 ±139	164 ±109 (7)
B-none	9.3 ±4.3	11.3 ±5.7	10.9 ±5.5 (29)	4.55 ±2.16	4.08 ±1.75	4.20 ±1.83 (33)	104 ±52	129 ±87	123 ±80 (33)
B-1	6.1 ±3.0	11.9 ±6.3	11.2 ±6.3 (25)	3.79 ±2.79	2.85 ±1.08	3.04 ±1.57 (40)	186 ±145	156 ±74	162 ±92 (39)
B-2	7.6 ±5.0	10.1 ±4.0	9.9 ±1.1 (51)	3.34 ±2.18	2.67 ±1.29	2.79 ±1.48 (39)	154 ±137	204 ±124	196 ±126 (37)
B-RP	12.3 ±10.3	8.0 ±3.7	10.0 ±7.7 (37)	3.50 ±2.51	3.82 ±2.63	3.73 ±2.57 (41)	167 ±118	165 ±138	165 ±131 (41)
P values†	P_1 0.001 P_2 0.001 S 0.05 IP_1 0.001 IP_2 0.01 SP 0.01 IS 0.025 ISP_1 0.01 ISP_2 0.025			P_1 0.05 P_2 0.06 S 0.05 IP_1 0.02			P_1 0.01		

S, supplemented; NS, nonsupplemented; Av, average. Number of subjects in parentheses.
*Raitman Frankel units per ml plasma on a basis of 45% hematocrit.
†See Table 13–3 for abbreviations.

Table 13–13. LEVELS OF ERYTHROCYTE AND SERUM FOLIC ACID AND SERUM VITAMIN B_{12} (MEAN ± SD) IN SUBJECTS USING ORAL CONTRACEPTIVES

	Erythrocyte folic acid (ng/ml)			Serum folic acid (ng/ml)			Serum vitamin B_{12} (pg/ml)		
	S	NS	Av	S	NS	Av	S	NS	Av
A-none	318 ±170	264 ±107	295 ±150 (102)	6.59 ±4.67	5.84 ±3.77	6.30 ±4.33 (107)	469 ±172	446 ±176	457 ±172 (28)
A-1	204 ±77	175 ±56	135 ±64 (28)	4.47 ±1.19	4.71 ±2.50	4.62 ±2.04 (18)	350 ±127	290 ±102	315 ±113 (17)
A-2	253 ±119	197 ±107	208 ±110 (36)	4.92 ±3.11	4.47 ±3.15	4.55 ±3.09 (27)	590 ±433	461 ±256	482 ±279 (19)
A-RP	457 ±313	260 ±165	430 ±304 (88)	7.72 ±5.86	5.89 ±5.23	7.50 ±5.79 (83)	435 ±173	679 ±642	464 ±273 (60)
B-none	230 ±81	181 ±73	192 ±77 (63)	4.20 ±1.93	3.34 ±1.24	3.53 ±1.45 (54)	416 ±72	521 ±232	499 ±212 (38)
B-1	222 ±160	200 ±91	204 ±107 (55)	4.41 ±3.48	4.02 ±1.64	4.09 ±2.01 (49)	385 ±125	378 ±221	380 ±204 (22)
B-2	199 ±83	172 ±65	176 ±69 (106)	4.79 ±2.18	3.84 ±1.30	3.96 ±1.45 (79)	487 ±201	478 ±270	479 ±259 (67)
B-RP	263 ±214	234 ±160	214 ±180 (82)	6.43 ±6.78	3.86 ±1.89	4.73 ±4.33 (72)	452 ±274	478 ±246	466 ±255 (36)
P Values*		P_2 0.001 I 0.001 S 0.001 IP_2 0.01			P_2 0.025			P_3 0.01	

*See Table 13–3 for abbreviations.
S, supplemented; NS, not supplemented; Av, average; number of subjects in parentheses.

Table 13–14. DUNCAN'S NEW MULTIPLE RANGE TEST* FOR ERYTHROCYTE AND SERUM FOLIC ACID IN ORAL CONTRACEPTIVE USERS (P <0.05)

	A-RP	A-none	B-RP	A-2	B-1	B-none	A-1	B-2
Erythrocyte folic acid (μg/ml)	430	295	244	208	204	192	185	176
	A-RP	A-none	B-RP	A-1	A-2	B-1	B-2	B-none
Serum folic acid (μg/ml)	7.50	6.30	4.7	4.6	4.55	4.09	3.96	3.53

*Any two means not underscored by the same line are significantly different. Any two means underscored by the same line are not significantly different.

DISCUSSION

It is obvious that subjects in the lower socioeconomic group showed a higher frequency of clinical signs indicative of malnutrition. Although the supplemented subjects in the higher socioeconomic group had less incidence of abnormal clinical findings related to nutrition, this was not observed in the other group. This may mean that subjects in the lower socioeconomic group either received inadequate supplements or falsely reported taking nutritional supplements.

In the higher socioeconomic group, greater frequencies of abnormal clinical signs, indicative of malnutrition, were observed in OCA users as compared to controls. However, this was not observed in subjects in the lower socioeconomic group taking OCA except for angular lesions of the mouth and debris or calculus of the teeth. An increase in incidences of dental caries in OCA users of the higher socioeconomic group was also observed. In rats injected with OCA, elevated incidences of carious lesions proportional to increased doses of OCA have been reported by Liu and Lin (38). Furthermore, these authors postulated that the increased dental caries activity of OCA-treated rats may be caused by a decrease in plasma zinc concentration, since such a reduction has been observed in human subjects (21, 55) and rats (35, 43) receiving OCA.

Increased levels of serum iron and TIBC due to OCA, as observed in our study, are consistent with the reports of other investigators who showed an increase in transferrin level due to OCA administration (6, 11, 25). Subjects resuming OCA after pregnancy in both groups appeared to be iron deficient as determined by serum iron and TIBC levels. We believe that changes in RP groups are a result of pregnancy and parturition and not due to OCA inasmuch as the subjects received OCA for a short period of time. The hemoglobin, hematocrit, and RBC count were, however, decreased only in the A-RP group; the explanation for a lack of similar finding in the B group is not apparent. In general, however, hypochromasia was present in group B, suggesting that iron deficiency was perhaps a complicating factor in that group.

The effect of OCA on plasma copper was similar to what has been reported (11, 12, 69). It is believed that this effect is mainly due to increased levels of ceruloplasmin in the plasma, which has been observed in OCA users and in pregnancy (12, 65).

With respect to effect of OCA on plasma zinc, conflicting data have been reported in the literature (6, 21, 50, 69). A significant decrease in plasma zinc levels as a result of OCA administration was reported by Halsted *et al.* (21), Briggs and Briggs (6), and Schenker *et al.* (69). O'Leary and Spellacy (50), however, reported an increase in the mean plasma zinc levels due to OCA. Their subjects received OCA for only 19 days, and the range of normal values was very wide (95–175 μg/100 ml). In addition, only 16 OCA users were used in their study. It is possible that small sample size and probable contamination problems in sample preparation may have contributed to their conflicting results.

Our studies indicate a significant decrease in plasma zinc levels but an increase in erythrocyte zinc content as a result of OCA administration. It is well known that estrogens increase plasma levels of several proteins such as ceruloplasmin, transferrin, thyroxine-binding globulin, and cortisol-binding protein (6, 12, 25). Inasmuch as over 80% of zinc in the red cells is bound to carbonic anhydrase apoenzyme (80), our data would suggest that synthesis or turnover of this protein may have been enhanced due to OCA. A similar effect was observed in RP groups, suggesting that the same estrogen effect due to pregnancy may have been present in these subjects. Further studies are indicated to document the specific effect of estrogen on the carbonic anhydrase turnover rate.

The mechanisms responsible for a decrease in plasma zinc levels remain to be elucidated. Several possibilities exist. Decreased absorption or increased excretion due to OCA may be responsible for such effect in the plasma. A redistribution of zinc between plasma and red cell pool should also be considered as another possible explanation. We have observed a decrease in serum albumin levels in OCA users. This protein is a major carrier for zinc (53), thus a decrease in plasma zinc may be related to a decrease in serum albumin levels. Another possibility is that serum albumin may have decreased in subjects using OCA due to a zinc-deficient state per se, as reported by Ronaghy *et al.* (62). At this stage, however, one cannot establish zinc deficiency in such subjects by plasma zinc level alone.

Gal *et al.* (20) reported a significant increase in vitamin A levels in the serum of patients using OCA as compared to their controls. Serum carotene levels, on the other hand, showed a decrease in OCA groups in comparison to the controls, when the serum sample was obtained between 18 to 21 days of the menstrual cycle. Our results are similar to those of Gal *et al.* (20). However, Yeung and Gillis (85) reported that, although plasma vitamin A levels may be increased as a result of the use of OCA in experimental animals, the liver content of vitamin A is decreased. Laurell *et al.* (33) has reported that a specific α-globulin responsible for binding vitamin A may be increased in the plasma, accounting for an increase in plasma vitamin A level. These results suggest that OCA effects mobilization and redistribution of tissue vitamin A stores and indeed the possibility that the vitamin A requirement may actually be increased due to OCA must be considered. Lowered levels of plasma carotene in OCA groups remains essentially unexplained.

Decreased ascorbic acid levels in platelets and leukocytes of women using OCA have been reported by some investigators (7, 27). Rivers and Devine (61) observed a decrease in plasma ascorbic acid levels in 4 women using OCA. In experimental animals, the lowered plasma vitamin C level is believed to be due to estrogens (68). Estrogen is known to induce adrenal hypertrophy and to reduce adrenal and plasma ascorbic acid levels, and ascorbic acid supplement reduces estrogen-induced adrenal hypertrophy in animals (15). Estrogen also induces hypophyseal hypertrophy and ascorbic acid depletion, and vitamin C administration depresses corticotrophic release (4).

The lower levels and higher rate of metabolism of ascorbic acid in the plasma, leukocytes, and platelets of women taking OCA may relate to their increased serum copper levels. Estrogens and OCA increase serum levels of copper and ceruloplasmin, the protein which transports copper. Ceruloplasmin catalyzes the oxidation of ascorbic acid *in vitro;* thus, it may participate in lowering ascorbic acid level in the plasma and tissues (23). We were, however, unable to document any change in plasma ascorbate levels due to OCA. Further studies are needed to determine whether or not ascorbate levels in the tissues is being affected in OCA users.

Most investigators believe that the requirement for vitamin B_6 is increased by estrogens (39, 63, 84). The estrogen effects in vitamin B_6 metabolism appear to occur in two ways. Firstly, estrogen increases the circulating levels of cortisol, which in turn increases the activity of tryptophan oxygenase (10). This enzyme is rate limiting in the pathway by which tryptophan is converted to niacin. Some of the enzymes in this pathway require vitamin B_6 as coenzymes, so that the requirement of vitamin B_6 is enhanced. Secondly, the metabolic products of estrogen and estrogen sulfate interfere with the binding of vitamin B_6 coenzymes to B_6-dependent enzymes, further increasing the requirement of vitamin B_6 for metabolic purposes.

The reduction in PLP level due to OCA was seen only in the upper socioeconomic group of subjects in this study. The subjects in the lower socioeconomic group did not show this effect. Furthermore, the reduction in EGOT activities due to OCA was greater in the lower than in the higher socioeconomic group of subjects. The activity of EGOT is dependent on the concentration of the coenzyme PLP. Addition of PLP to the assay mixture increases the activity of the EGOT. The activation is related inversely to the concentration of PLP in the red cells and so may serve as an additional indicator of vitamin B_6 status of the subjects. The percent stimulation of EGOT was higher in the OCA and RP subjects in both socioeconomic groups in our study, suggesting a relative deficiency of the vitamin in these subjects. This may indicate that the EGOT stimulation test is a more sensitive index of alterations in vitamin B_6 status than plasma PLP or EGOT measurements.

Impairment of glucose tolerance is an important abnormality found in some OCA users which may be related to vitamin B_6 deficiency. Increased resistance to insulin by peripheral tissues, such as parametrial adipose tissues and diaphragm muscle *in vitro* and *in vivo,* was found to be responsible for the impairment of glucose tolerance in experimental animals treated with OCA (36, 37). Murakami (46) suggested that xanthurenic acid is capable of complexing with insulin, thereby reducing its biologic activity. A significant reduction in biologic activity of the insulin in the complex was observed by means of rat diaphragm and epididymal fat pad bioassays (46), and a 50% reduction in the hypoglycemic effect of the insulin was observed when the complex was injected into dogs and rabbits (28, 29). Indeed, a small group of women whose carbohydrate tolerance had become impaired while taking OCA improved after vitamin B_6 administration. Several investigators have suggested that large doses of vitamin B_6 should be added to OCA indiscriminately. However, Adams *et al.* (1) indicated that the administration of coenzyme may increase apoenzyme synthesis and that this may enhance the plasma-amino-acid-lowering effect of OCA, which may have an untoward effect in communities where protein malnutrition exists. At present, it would appear that the idea of supplementation of vitamin B_6 should be approached cautiously, since the long-term effect of such therapy is uncertain.

Folic acid metabolism is altered by orally administered estrogen, but the nature and significance of this alteration is not clear. Several isolated cases of OCA users evidencing clinical signs of folate deficiency have been described (26, 51, 66, 67). In all these cases, the dietary intake has been adequate to good, and generally the women were considered to be healthy. Masked malabsorption or occult malabsorption has been implicated as the underlying cause for the folic acid deficiency and severe megaloblastic anemia in some cases.

Conflicting data have been published with respect to serum folate levels in OCA users. However, the majority of reports indicate a decrease in serum folate at least in some of the subjects using OCA (70, 71, 81). Red cell folate also decreased and FIGLU excretion following histidine loading has been observed to increase in OCA users (40). These abnormalities are corrected following folic acid supplementation.

Streiff (76) and Necheles and Snyder (48) suggested that there is an oral-estrogen-induced impairment to the hydrolysis of the complex folic acid polyglutamate which leads to poor absorption of dietary folate. Later studies of Stephens et al. (75) and Shojania et al. (72), however, indicated that the absorption of the polyglutamate form of folic acid may not be impaired but that folate metabolism is significantly altered in OCA users. According to Stephens et al. (75) the absorption of the polyglutamic folic acid was similar to that of monoglutamic folic acid in OCA users, provided that these subjects were saturated with folic acid prior to the study. These results suggest an alteration in the rate of folic acid uptake or metabolism by the tissues. In experimental animals, oral sex hormones increase the activities of intestinal enzymes involved in folate metabolism, suggesting that estrogens may increase the rate of metabolism of folic acid and its metabolites by the intestine. The most significant result of the modified folic acid metabolism of women taking OCA may be the possible depletion of body stores of folic acid. Since many of the women discontinue OCA to conceive, Pritchard et al. (57) have suggested that the women becoming pregnant soon after discontinuing the pill may have a high chance of developing folic acid deficiency during pregnancy.

Recently, a protein which binds unreduced folates and dihydrofolate has been identified in leukocyte lysates and serum from some women taking OCA (16). It has been suggested that with inadequate or marginal intake of folate, the hormonal induction of this protein may contribute to megaloblastosis by sequestering dihydrofolate and the intermediary folate coenzyme in DNA-thymine synthesis.

Our results show a definite lowering effect of OCA on red cell folate concentrations in subjects of the upper socioeconomic group. In the lower socioeconomic group, both the plasma and red cell folate levels were lower than in the upper socioeconomic group of subjects, indicating that this population may be marginally deficient in folic acid. Our data are consistent with the hypothesis that the subjects in the lower socioeconomic group were marginally deficient in several micronutrients and that this may have been responsible for a difference in the effects of OCA on several parameters in this group of subjects as compared to the upper socioeconomic group. Further studies are needed to clarify the clinical significance of these differences with respect to the effect of OCA in the two groups of subjects.

CONCLUSION

The epidemiologic aspects of OCA on nutrient metabolism were studied in a large population of women. Incidence of clinical abnormalities related to malnutrition were more frequently observed in the lower (B) as compared to the higher (A) socioeconomic groups. In the A groups some clinical signs were more common in the nonsupplemented groups of subjects. In general, the intake of OCA subjects for calories, protein, calcium, magnesium, iron, copper, and zinc did not differ from that of the controls. The intake of the above nutrients in group A subjects were higher than those of group B except for calories. The subjects who took supplements had higher intakes of calcium, iron, magnesium, and copper. No effect of OCA was seen on hemoglobin, hematocrit, or erythrocyte count. The levels of serum iron were increased due to Norinyl. Total iron-binding capacity was increased as a result of OCA administration; TIBC values were higher in group B as compared to group A and in the nonsupplemented as compared to the supplemented groups. Plasma copper levels were increased and plasma zinc levels were decreased as a result of OCA administration. An increase in erythrocyte zinc concentrations was observed due to Norinyl. No effect of OCA on levels of plasma calcium and magnesium and erythrocyte magnesium was observed. Although no effect of OCA on plasma total protein was found, the level of serum albumin was decreased.

As a rule, the intake of OCA subjects of vitamin A and C did not differ from that of the controls. As expected, subjects from the supplemented groups had higher intake of vitamin A, C, thiamine, and riboflavin, and A groups had a higher intake of vitamin C and riboflavin.

Increased plasma vitamin A and decreased carotene levels were observed in OCA users. In general, OCA had little or no effect on plasma ascorbic acid levels. Urinary excretion of both thiamine and riboflavin in subjects using OCA were lower in A groups. Subjects who took supplements had higher levels of plasma vitamin A and ascorbic acid, but levels of urinary thiamine and riboflavin were higher only in group A subjects who took supplements.

Dietary intake of vitamin B_6 and folic acid by OCA subjects did not differ from that of controls, although, in general, subjects in the A group had higher intake of vitamin B_6 and folic acid than those in the B group. Subjects from the supplemented groups had higher intake of vitamin B_6 and folic acid in comparison to the nonsupplemented groups. In group A, higher intake of vitamin B_6 and folic acid was observed in subjects resuming the pill (RP) as compared to the subjects using OCA. Plasma PLP and red cell and serum folate levels were lower in OCA subjects in group A as compared to the controls. Reduction in EGOT activity and elevation in the EGOT stimulation test were observed in OCA subjects in both groups (A and B). These observations suggest a relatively deficient state with respect to B_6 and folic acid in OCA users. No significant effect on serum vitamin B_{12} was observed as a result of OCA administration.

CHANGES IN LEVELS OF PLASMA IRON, COPPER, AND ZINC DUE TO PREGNANCY

Only a few reports are available in the literature concerning changes in trace elements as a result of pregnancy. These will be summarized here.

Iron deficiency anemia ranging in incidence from 15% (2) to 58% (56) has been observed in pregnant women as reported from the United States. A rise in serum iron (32, 42) and total iron-binding capacity (32) during pregnancy have been reported by many investigators. This rise in TIBC is probably independent of iron deficiency and can occur without alterations in serum iron or hemoglobin (45). Thus, the elevation of TIBC in late pregnancy, like that which occurs much more rapidly in women on oral contraceptive agents, appeared to be hormonal in origin. In early pregnancy a rise in serum iron—but not in TIBC—which cannot therefore be secondary to a rise in TIBC has been reported (32, 42, 77). A shift of inorganic iron from body stores to extracellular fluid would seem most likely to be the explanation for the rise in serum iron. Hemoglobin levels normally fall in the third trimester of pregnancy due partly to an increase in plasma volume and partly to increased requirement of iron during pregnancy. Supplemental iron significantly increased hemoglobin levels but had no effect upon the hydremia of the pregnancy (18).

In a study of 31 pregnant women, Nielsen (49) found serum copper to increase from the third month to an average of 2.7 µg/ml, compared with a normal nonpregnant level of 1.2 µg/ml. Various investigators (19, 21, 30, 64) have also reported similar results. In these studies, the red cell copper remained at normal levels throughout pregnancy. The high serum copper level of pregnancy returns to normal in the first few weeks postpartum (19).

As exogenous estrogens are known to raise both serum copper and ceruloplasmin levels (65), it has been thought that the increase observed during pregnancy is due to increased endogenous estrogens.

Halsted et al. (21) reported a reduction of plasma zinc levels for 25 women in the third trimester of pregnancy. In addition, O'Leary and Spellacy (50) reported a similar trend in 30 pregnant women. These reports indicate that changes in the plasma levels of iron, copper, and zinc in pregnancy are quite similar to those reported in women taking OCA. The mechanisms and physiologic importance of these changes remain unknown at present and clearly further investigations are needed in this area.

ACKNOWLEDGMENTS

We gratefully acknowledge the technical help of Elizabeth Bowersox, Kay Lord, Elizabeth DuMouchelle, Daria Koniuch, Jim Nowak, Ray Collins, and Virginia Kortes.

Plasma pyridoxal phosphate determinations were performed in the laboratory of Dr. Paul Gyorgy and Dr. Catherine Rose in Philadelphia, and folate determinations were done in the laboratory of Dr. Jack Smith, Dr. Jeff Lawrence, and Dr. Grace Goldsmith in New Orleans. We wish to express our appreciation for their help.

REFERENCES

1. Adams PW, Wynn V, Rose DP, Folkard J, Seed M, Strong R: Effect of pyridoxine hydrochloride (Vitamin B_6) upon depression associated with oral contraception. Lancet 1:897, 1973
2. Allaire BI, Campagna FA: Iron-deficiency anemia in pregnancy. Evaluation of diagnosis and therapy by bone marrow hemosiderin. Obstet Gynecol 17:605, 1961
3. Aly HE, Donald EA, Simpson MHW: Oral contraceptives and vitamin B_6 metabolism. Am J Clin Nutr 24:297, 1971
4. Bacchus H, Altszuler N: Eosinophil response to stress in ascorbic acid pretreated mice. Endocrinology 51:1, 1952
5. Bianchine JR, Bonnlander B, Macaraeg PVJ, Hersey R, Bianchine JW, McIntyre PA: Serum vitamin B_{12} binding capacity and oral contraceptive hormones. J Clin Endocrinol Metab 29:1425, 1969
6. Briggs MH, Briggs M: Contraceptives and serum proteins. Br Med J 3:521, 1970
7. Briggs M, Briggs M: Vitamin C requirements and oral contraceptives. Nature [New Biol] 238:277, 1972
8. Briggs MH, Pitchford AG, Staniford M, Barker HM, Taylor D: Metabolic effects of steroid contraceptives. Steroid Biochem Pharm 2:111, 1970
9. Brown RR, Rose DP, Leklem JE, Linkswiler H, Anand R: Urinary 4-pyridoxic acid, plasma pyridoxal phosphate, and erythrocyte aminotransferase levels in oral contraceptive users receiving controlled intakes of vitamin B_6. Am J Clin Nutr 28:10, 1975
10. Bulbrook RD, Hayward JL, Herian M, Swain MC, Tong D, Wang DY: Effect of steroidal contraceptives on levels of plasma androgen sulphates and cortisol. Lancet 1:628, 1973
11. Burton JL: Effect of oral contraceptives on haemoglobin, packed-cell volume, serum-iron and total iron-binding capacity in healthy women. Lancet 1:978, 1967
12. Carruthers ME, Hobbs CB, Warren RL: Raised serum copper and caeruloplasmin levels in subjects taking oral contraceptives. J Clin Pathol 19:498, 1966
13. Castren OM, Rossi RR: Effect of oral contraceptives on serum folic acid content. J Obstet Gynaecol Br Commonw 77:548, 1970
14. Chabner BA, Livingston DM: A simple enzymic assay for pyridoxal phosphate. Anal Biochem 34:413, 1970
15. Chatterjee A, Bardhan NR: The influence of ascorbic acid on the rat adrenal in stilbestrol induced stress. Naturwissenschaften 53:110, 1966
16. DaCosta M, Rothenberg SP: Appearance of a folate binder in leukocytes and serum of women who are pregnant or taking oral contraceptives. J Lab Clin Med 83:207, 1974
17. Davis RE, Smith BK: Pyridoxal, vitamin B_{12} and folate metabolism in women taking oral contraceptive agents. S Afr Med J 48:1937, 1974

18. deLeeuw NK, Lowenstein L, Hsieh YS: Iron deficiency and hydremia in normal pregnancy. Medicine (Baltimore) 45:291, 1966
19. Fay J, Cartwright GE, Wintrobe MM: Studies on free erythrocyte protoporphyrin, serum iron, serum iron-binding capacity and plasma copper during normal pregnancy. J Clin Invest 28:487, 1949
20. Gal I, Parkinson C, Craft I: Effects of oral contraceptives on human plasma vitamin-A levels. Br Med J 2:436, 1971
21. Halsted JA, Hackley BM, Smith JC: Plasma zinc and copper in pregnancy and after oral contraceptives. Lancet 2:278, 1968
22. Hontz AC, Gyorgy P, Balin H, Rose CS, Shaw DL: Interaction of contraceptive steroids with metabolic functions of vitamin B_6 (abstr). Am J Clin Nutr 27:440, 1974
23. Humoller FL, Mockler MP, Holthaus JM, Mahler DJ: Enzymatic properties of ceruloplasmin. J Lab Clin Med 56:222, 1960
24. Interdepartment Committee on Nutrition for National Defense: Manual for Nutrition Surveys, 2nd ed. Bethesda, National Institutes of Health, 1963
25. Jacobi JM, Powell LW, Gaffney TJ: Immunochemical quantitation of human transferrin in pregnancy and during the administration of oral contraceptives. Br J Haematol 17:503, 1969
26. Johnson GK, Geenan JE, Hensley GT, Soergel KH: Small intestinal disease, folate deficiency anemia, and oral contraceptive agents. Am J Dig Dis 18:185, 1973
27. Kalesh DG, Mallikarjuneswara VR, Clemetson CAB: Effect of estrogen-containing oral contraceptives on platelet and plasma ascorbic acid concentrations. Contraception 4:183, 1971
28. Kotake Y, Sotokawa T, Murakami E, Hisatake A, Abe M, Ikeda Y: Studies on the xanthurenic acid-insulin complex. II. Physiological activities. J Biochem 63:578, 1968
29. Kotake Y, Sotokawa T, Murakami E, Hisatake A, Abe M, Ikeda Y: Physiological activities of xanthurenic acid-8 methyl ether-insulin complex. J Biochem 64:895, 1968
30. Krebs HA: Über das Kupfer im menschlichen Blutserum. Klin Wochenschr 7:584, 1928
31. Larsson–Cohn U: An appraisal of the clinical effect of three different oral contraceptive agents and their influence on transaminase activity. Acta Obstet Gynecol Scand 45:499, 1966
32. Laurell CB: Studies on transportation and metabolism of iron in body, with special reference to iron-binding component in human plasma. Acta Physiol Scand [Suppl] 14(46):1, 1947
33. Laurell CB, Kullander S, Thorell J: Effect of administration of a combined estrogen-progestin contraceptive on the level of individual plasma proteins. Scand J Clin Lab Invest 21:337, 1968
34. Lawrence J: Personal communication from Touro Research Institute, Biochemistry Research, New Orleans, LA 70115
35. Lei KY, Prasad AS, Bowersox E, Oberleas D: Oral contraceptives, norethindrone and mestranol: effect on zinc and copper metabolism. Fed Proc 34:922, 1975
36. Lei KY, Yang MG: Oral contraceptives, norethynodrel and mestranol: effects on glucose tolerance, tissue uptake of glucose-U-^{14}C and insulin sensitivity. Proc Soc Exp Biol Med 141:130, 1972
37. Lei KY, Yang MG, Oberleas D, Prasad AS: Oral contraceptives: effects on plasma insulin response to glucose and on the response to insulin and 2-deoxyglucose uptake by peripheral tissue. Proc Soc Exp Biol Med 149:417, 1975
38. Liu FTY, Lin HS: Effect of the contraceptive steroids norethynodrel and mestranol on dental caries activity in young adult female rats. J Dent Res 52:753, 1973
39. Luhby AL, Reyniak JV, Brin M, Sambour M, Brin H: Abnormal vitamin B_6 metabolism in menopausal women given estrogenic steroids and its correction by pyridoxine. Am J Clin Nutr 26:468, 1973

40. Luhby AL, Shimizu N, Davis P, Copperman JM: Folic acid deficiency in users of oral contraceptive agents. Fed Proc 30:239, 1971
41. Lumeng L, Cleary RE, Li TK: Effect of oral contraceptives on the plasma concentration of pyridoxal phosphate. Am J Clin Nutr 27:326, 1974
42. Mardell M, Symons C, Zilva JF: A comparison of the effect of oral contraceptives, pregnancy and sex on iron metabolism. J Clin Endocrinol Metab 29:1489, 1969
43. McBean LD, Smith JC, Halsted JA: Effect of oral contraceptive hormones on zinc metabolism in the rat. Proc Soc Exp Biol Med 137:543, 1971
44. McLean FW, Heine MW, Held B, Streiff RR: Relationship between the oral contraceptive and folic acid metabolism. Am J Obstet Gynecol 104:745, 1969
45. Morgan EH: Plasma-iron and haemoglobin levels in pregnancy. The effect of oral iron. Lancet 1:9, 1961
46. Murakami E: Studies on the xanthurenic acid-insulin complex. I. Preparation and properties. J Biochem 63:573, 1968
47. Myrianthopoulos NC, French K: An application of the U.S. Bureau of the Census Socioeconomic Index to a large, diversified patient population. Soc Sci Med 2:283, 1968
48. Necheles TF, Snyder LM: Malabsorption of folate polyglutamates associated with oral contraceptive therapy. N Engl J Med 282: 858, 1970
49. Nielsen AL: On serum copper; normal values. Acta Med Scand 118:87, 1944
50. O'Leary JA, Spellacy WN: Zinc and copper levels in pregnant women and those taking oral contraceptives. Am J Obstet Gynecol 103:131, 1969
51. Paton AL: Oral contraceptives and folate deficiency. Lancet 1:418, 1969
52. Prasad AS, Lei KY, Oberleas D, Moghissi KS, Stryker JC: Effect of oral contraceptive agents on nutrients. II. Vitamins. Am J Clin Nutr 28:385, 1975
53. Prasad AS, Oberleas D: Binding of zinc to amino acids and serum proteins in vitro. J Lab Clin Med 76:416, 1970
54. Prasad AS, Oberleas D, Halsted JA: Determination of zinc in biological fluids by atomic absorption spectrophotometry. In Prasad AS (ed): Zinc Metabolism. Springfield, Ill, C Thomas, 1966, pp 27–37
55. Prasad AS, Oberleas D, Lei KY, Moghissi KS, Stryker JC: Effect of oral contraceptive agents on nutrients. I. Minerals. Am J Clin Nutr 28:377, 1975
56. Pritchard JA, Hunt CF: A comparison of the hemetologic responses following the routine prenatal administration of intramuscular and oral iron. Surg Gynecol Obstet 106:516, 1958
57. Pritchard JA, Scott DE, Whalley PJ: Maternal folate deficiency and pregnancy wastage. IV. Effects of folic acid supplements, anticonvulsants and oral contraceptives. Am J Obstet Gynecol 109:341, 1971
58. Raica N, Sauberlich HE: Blood cell transaminase activity in human vitamin B_6 deficiency. Am J Clin Nutr 15:67, 1964
59. Reitman S, Frankel S: A colorimetric method for the determination of serum glutamic oxalacetic and glutamic pyruvic transaminases. Am J Clin Pathol 28:56, 1967
60. Riggs BL, Jowsey J, Kelly PJ, Jones JHD, Maher FT: Effect of sex hormones on bone in primary osteoporosis. J Clin Invest 48:1065, 1969
61. Rivers JM, Devine MM: Plasma ascorbic acid concentrations and oral contraceptives. Am J Clin Nutr 25:684, 1972
62. Ronaghy HA, Reinhold JG, Mahloudji M, Ghavami P, Spivey–Fox MR, Halsted JA: Zinc supplementation of malnourished schoolboys in Iran: increased growth and other effects. Am J Clin Nutr 27:112, 1974
63. Rose DP: The influence of oestrogens on tryptophan metabolism in man. Clin Sci 31:265, 1966
64. Rottger H: Kupfer bei Mutter und Kind. (Copper in mother and child). Arch Gynaekol 177:650, 1950

65. Russ EM, Raymunt J: Influence of estrogens on total serum copper and caeruloplasmin. Proc Soc Exp Biol Med 92:465, 1956
66. Ryser JE, Farquet JJ, Petite J: Megaloblastic anemia due to folic acid deficiency in a young woman on oral contraceptives. Acta Haematol 45:319, 1971
67. Salter WM: Megaloblastic anemia and oral contraceptives. Minn Med 55:554, 1972
68. Saroja N, Mallikarjuneswara VR, Clemetson CAB: Effect of estrogens on ascorbic acid in the plasma and blood vessels of guinea pigs. Contraception 3:269, 1971
69. Schenker JG, Hellerstein S, Jungreis E, Polishuk WZ: Serum copper and zinc levels in patients taking oral contraceptives. Fertil Steril 22:229, 1971
70. Shojania AM, Hornady GJ, Barnes PH: Oral contraceptives and serum folate level. Lancet 1:1376, 1968
71. Shojania AM, Hornady GJ, Barnes PH: Oral contraceptives and folate metabolism. Lancet 1:886, 1969
72. Shojania AM, Hornady GJ, Barnes PH: The effect of oral contraceptives on folate metabolism. Am J Obstet Gynecol 111:782, 1971
73. Simpson GR, Dale E: Serum levels of phosphorus, magnesium and calcium in women utilizing combination oral or long-acting injectable progestational contraceptives. Fertil Steril 23:326, 1972
74. Skeggs HR: Vitamin B_{12}. In Gyorgy P, Pearson WN (eds): The Vitamins, Vol 7. New York, Academic Press, 1967, pp 277–293
75. Stephens MEN, Craft I, Peters TJ, Hoffbrand AV: Oral contraceptives and folate metabolism. Clin Sci 42:405, 1972
76. Streiff RR: Folate deficiency and oral contraceptives. JAMA 214:105, 1970
77. Sturegon P: Studies of iron requirements in infants. III. Influence of supplemental iron during normal pregnancy on mother and infant. A. The mother. Br J Haematol 5:31, 1959
78. Technicon Auto-Analyzer Methodology. Technicon Instrument Corp, Tarrytown, New York 10591, 1972
79. Theuer RC: Effect of oral contraceptive agents on vitamin and mineral needs: a review. J Reprod Med 8:13, 1972
80. Vallee BL: Biochemistry, physiology and pathology of zinc. Physiol Rev 39:443, 1959
81. Wertalik LF, Metz EN, Lobuglio AF, Balcerzak SP: Decreased serum B_{12} levels with oral contraceptive use. JAMA 221:1371, 1972
82. Winer BJ: Statistical Principles in Experimental Design. New York, McGraw–Hill, 1962
83. Wintrobe MM: Clinical Hematology, 6th ed. Philadelphia, Lea & Febiger, 1967
84. Wolf H, Brown RR, Price JM, Madsen PO: Studies on tryptophan metabolism in male subjects treated with female sex hormones. J Clin Endocrinol Metab 31:397, 1970
85. Yeung DL, Gillis C: Oral contraceptives and vitamin A (abstr). IX Int Congr Nutr Amsterdam, Exerpta Medica, 1972, p 21
86. Zip Zone Serum Protein Electrophoresis Procedure: Procedure 1. Helena Laboratories, Beaumont, TX 1973

Chapter 14

Hormonal Contraception and Nutrition

Mark A. Belsey

In the absence of a specific disease state, no other medication or drug is used as widely and continuously, and for such prolonged periods, as hormonal contraceptives.

Hormonal contraceptives are widely used in the family planning programs of developing countries. The diets of women in both rural and urban areas are often deficient, particularly in proteins, many vitamins, and some minerals. Often health services in these countries are insufficient and unable to maintain close individualized supervision on all women, including those considered to be at high risk of developing complications. Many of these women suffer from a variety of endemic diseases that may affect their nutritional status and their capacity to metabolize exogenous hormonal steroids.

Yet, despite such widespread use, our knowledge of the health consequences of the interaction of hormonal contraception and nutrition is limited. Published research on the subject, other than that related to vitamin and mineral metabolism, is almost nil; few reports have dealt with the problem of hormonal contraception in nutritionally deficient women. This chapter poses more questions than answers.

At present, the potential interaction between nutrition and hormonal contraception can be inferred either from clinical studies on the metabolic effects of hormonal contraceptives or from epidemiologic studies of risk factors known to be associated with the nutritional status of a woman.

In discussing nutritional interaction with hormonal contraception from a metabolic perspective, the changes in carbohydrate, lipid, and protein metabolism will be considered. The effect of nutrition on some of these metabolic changes is problematic. In discussing the clinical implications of the interaction between nutrition and hormonal contraception, we assume a link between nutrition and the metabolic changes and the clinical conditions that are increasingly associated with the use of hormonal contraceptives.

For example, diet is a major factor affecting blood lipid levels and obesity. Furthermore, at least epidemiologically, there is a clear association of blood cholesterol and obesity with the risk of occlusive cardiovascular disease. Hormonal contraceptives are associated with increased serum lipids and with increased risk of certain vascular diseases. Whether or not, or to what degree, such associations are in turn affected by nutrition is unknown. The influence of nutrition on the link between hormonal contraception and metabolic changes has not been examined by researchers. Similarly, the influence of nutrition on the link between hormonal contraception and clinical side effects and complications has not been examined, nor has the link between metabolic changes and clinical complications been clearly established.

Many of the therapeutic agents that have been developed for specific diseases are known to affect and to be affected by the nutritional state of the user. Furthermore, therapeutic agents may be metabolized differently in different racial groups and different individuals, depending on the presence and levels of specific enzymes in these groups or individuals. Certain drugs affect nutrition by affecting intestinal absorption or by competing with enzymes crucial for normal metabolism. Vitamin B_6 supplementation has become routine in the therapy for tuberculosis due to the competition of the enzyme in the acetylation of isoniazid. Such supplementation is essential to avoid serious deficiency disease in malnourished patients with tuberculosis.

Some of the effects of hormonal contraceptives on carbohydrate, lipid, and protein metabolism in healthy women in developed countries have been known for many years. The available data have been reviewed by scientific groups and published by the World Health Organization in its technical report series (12, 13). More recently, data have been accumulating on the effect of hormonal contraception on vitamin and mineral metabolism. These data have been summarized in several review articles (11, 16), in the most recent scientific group technical report on the subject (15), and in this book. But the existing information on the metabolic effects and clinical implications of hormonal contraception has been derived almost exclusively from studies performed in developed countries, on women with access to reasonably healthy diets and to a range of health services. The applicability of this information to women with a range of nutritional disorders or marginal deficiencies remains to be established.

The metabolic effects of hormonal contraception may be manifest by altered levels of the nutrient, its metabolites, and/or other metabolites or enzymes critically affected by the changed level or biologic activity of the nutrient. However, some of these changes may be of no clinical significance, but merely represent a change in the level of some substances. For example, the consistent reports of increased serum levels of vitamin A among oral contraceptive users is thought to represent a shift from tissue stores and not thought to be of the magnitude of concern in terms of increased vitamin A. If, however, the increased levels of vitamin A represent a shift from tissue to serum, the question may be asked as to whether such a shift results in tissue depletion in women whose vitamin A intake is marginal or deficient.

Some metabolic changes brought on or aggravated by oral contraceptives have a clear deleterious effect. For example, those rare individuals with congenital hyperlipidemia who use hormonal contraceptives are at greater risk of developing acute vascular accident.

Other effects may be advantageous to the user. Thus the indirect affect of decreased blood loss associated with hormonal contraception should result in increased hemoglobin and hematocrit. Similarly, though not known to be related to nutrition or metabolic activity, the decrease in benign breast tumors would be advantageous.

Finally, other metabolic effects are observed but are not clearly associated with clinical changes. Thus the plasma renin concentration, plasma renin substrate, and angiotensin II levels are increased in oral contraceptive users, regardless of whether hypertension develops or not.

The majority of observed metabolic effects have not been assessed in terms of their long-term health consequences. Thus, one can pose the following questions, which are further complicated by asking what role nutrition has on these potential long-term consequences: 1) What relationship exists between altered glucose metabolism, as expressed by an abnormal glucose tolerance test, and the risk of diabetes? 2) What are the long-term effects of elevated plasma triglycerides on the vascular tree? 3) Does prolonged elevation of the "carrier" proteins such as cortisol-binding globulin, transferrin, ceruloplasmin, and thyroid-binding globulin have an impact on health? 4) Does a rise of plasma renin concentration, plasma renin substrate, angiotensin II, etc. and a rise of 10–15 mm Hg in systolic blood pressure or 5–10 mm Hg in diastolic blood pressure have any clinical significance?

A discussion of the interaction of hormonal contraceptives and nutrition is complicated by the variety of preparations in use and the widely different metabolic effects particularly of the different progestogens. These preparations include combinations of different estrogens and progestogens, varying in dose, sequence and combination of use. Some of the apparent discrepancies in the reported metabolic effects of oral contraceptive agents may be attributable to the dosage, frequency, and duration of administration, in addition to the differences in the progestogen.

The health consequences of hormonal contraceptives is greatly affected by certain characteristics of the user, some of which are related to nutrition. Obesity and weight gain, clearly nutrition related, are important risk factors in a number of complications and side effects, including hypertension and abnormal glucose metabolism.

Many of the chronic diseases themselves interact with the nutrition of a woman. Tuberculosis is a well-known example of the deleterious interaction with undernutrition. One recent report from India suggests a beneficial effect of hormonal contraceptives (6). When used with adequate antituberculosis therapy, hormonal contraceptives are associated with an improved rate of recovery from the tuberculosis. In contrast, research performed for a doctoral dissertation in Egypt suggests that hormonal contraception may have a deleterious effect on liver function in the presence of schistosomiasis (9). This latter effect is influenced by the dosage of the contraceptive and the duration and severity of the schistosomiasis.

The disease–hormonal contraception interaction model of schistosomiasis is a rather useful example if confirmed. Liver damage, such as produced by schistosomiasis or secondary nutritional deficiency, is likely to be an important factor associated with adverse metabolic effects of hormonal contraceptives. In contrast to schistosomiasis, liver fluke infection *(Opisthorchis viverrini)* in Thailand is not associated with significant hepatocellular injury and does not appear to be associated with any significant differences in the metabolic effects when compared with the effects seen in uninfected women (14).

The role of the liver in understanding the interaction between nutrition and hormonal contraception is rather critical. It has been suggested that, in healthy women, only the plasma proteins produced in the liver are affected by oral hormonal contraceptives. Plasma proteins such as the immunoglobulins produced outside the liver appear unaffected. However, in the report on Oral Contraceptives and Health by the Royal College of General Practitioners (1) and in earlier reports from India (3) there is some suggestion of an affect of hormonal contraceptives on the immune response. These are potential but unproven risks of hormonal contraceptive use by women who have the pathologic changes associated with protein deficiency, particularly when such changes may be coupled with hepatocellular destruction from endemic hepatitis and parasitic infections involving the liver.

EFFECT OF HORMONAL CONTRACEPTION ON CARBOHYDRATE METABOLISM

A variable effect on carbohydrate metabolism has been noted. The effect is most often seen with combination estrogen-progestogen preparations but appears to be dependent on the specific progestogen. It has also been noted in women on long-acting injectable progestogen preparations, but this observation requires further confirmation. In healthy women there is an increase in the frequency of abnormal glucose tolerance tests (GTT), there may be a slight rise in the fasting blood sugar, and both plasma insulin and human growth hormone levels are elevated. The probability of an abnormal GTT developing in the course of oral hormonal contraception is increased when there has been a history of previous abnormal glucose metabolism, a family history of diabetes, delivery of an excessively large infant, obesity or excessive weight gain, or among older women with high parity.

An abnormal GTT is found in about 10 or 11% of women who have taken hormonal contraceptives for 1 year. The abnormal GTT appears reversible within 3 months of discontinuation.

There is reasonable evidence that the impairment of glucose metabolism in many women may be associated with the alteration of tryptophan metabolism and either a relative or absolute vitamin B_6 deficiency. Estrogens along with glucocorticoids have been noted to enhance the metabolism of tryptophan via the niacin pathway. Several of the enzyme reactions involved in the metabolism of tryptophan require pyridoxal phosphate as coenzyme, the coenzyme form of vitamin B_6. The decreased levels of vitamin B_6 associated with its increased requirement is coupled with a rise in the urinary excretion of several of the products of the increased tryptophan metabolism, including kynurenine, 3-hydroxykynurenine, and xanthurenic acid (Figure 14–1). It has been hypothesized that xanthurenic acid may bind to insulin and decrease its biologic activity.

The administration of vitamin B_6 in doses two to three times the daily requirement to women who have developed an abnormal GTT while receiving hormonal steroids has been found to improve their glucose tolerance (10). Similar results have been found in a number of women who developed gestational diabetes (3). In the latter study the women were also shown to have signs of pyridoxine deficiency with increased level of urinary xanthurenic acid. Pyridoxine administration resulted in a decrease in the urinary excretion of xanthurenic acid and a return to normal GTT in 12 of 14 women.

An alternative mechanism, enzyme induction and glyconeogenesis, has been postulated for those women who develop an abnormal GTT in the absence of evidence of vitamin B_6 deficiency and to account for the changes seen in the woman deficient in vitamin B_6 (16).

It has been suggested that the abnormal glucose metabolism in those without a vitamin B_6 deficiency may be due to estrogen-mediated glucocorticoid activity following induction of a number of pyridoxal phosphate-dependent enzymes, including alanine and tyrosine aminotransferase. The effect on glucose metabolism in vitamin B_6 deficiency might be due to gluconeogenesis. A reduction of quinolinic acid with decreased pyridoxal phosphate would result in increased phosphoenolpyruvate carboxykinase in the liver, since quinolinic acid has a limiting affect on the latter enzyme. Increased gluconeogenesis would occur as a result of the increased phosphoenolpyruvate carboxykinase activity.

Although neither mechanism—either via xanthenuric acid binding to insulin, or enzyme induction and glyconeogenesis—has been established, a word of caution has been raised in automatically assuming that vitamin B_6 supplementa-

Fig. 14–1. Tryptophan–nicotinamide metabolism pathway.

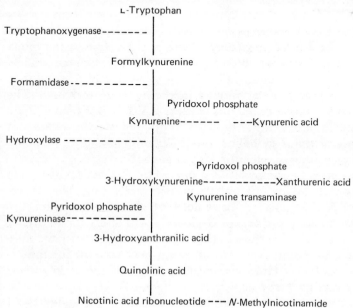

tion should be provided with estrogen-progestogen preparations (16). As discussed later on, total plasma amino acid levels fall in women on oral hormonal contraceptives. If vitamin B_6 supplements were given to women receiving hormonal contraceptives, it is possible that the coenzyme induction of apoenzyme could enhance the plasma amino acid lowering action of the estrogen, the clinical implications of which are unknown, particularly in women with protein malnutrition. Specific studies on vitamin B_6 supplementation would be required in communities where protein deficiency is not uncommon.

Although it has been thought that diabetes is less common in developing tropical and subtropical countries, available population surveys indicate that it is no less frequent than in many developed countries when based upon fasting blood glucose or on a 1-hour or 2-hour blood sugar level following a glucose load. There are currently no data available on glucose metabolism and hormonal contraception from developing countries.

Limited experimental studies using a small number of monkeys on a normal or a protein-deficient diet and receiving hormonal contraceptives have been undertaken in India but have been inconclusive (7). There was a slight but not particularly significant delay in the return of blood glucose to fasting levels, particularly in animals receiving the full protein diet, and only a marginal effect of hormonal contraceptives on the GTT in animals on the low-protein diet. The applicability of these results to malnutrition in women is uncertain.

A possible role of altered nutritional status may explain a recent finding of an accelerated return to fasting glucose blood levels found among Thai women receiving depomedroxyprogesterone acetate (DMPA). No such effect has been observed among women in developed countries.

PROTEIN METABOLISM

The effect of hormonal contraceptives on protein metabolism appears to be similar to the effect seen during pregnancy. There is a decrease in the blood levels of the amino acids proline, glycine, lysine, histidine, alanine, valine, tyrosine, and ornithine. Levels of serum albumin are generally decreased, while those of many of the other proteins formed in the liver are increased. The concentrations of blood coagulation factors (factors I, VII, VIII, IX, and X) are increased; concentrations of the carrier proteins mentioned previously are also increased, as are those of the β-globulins, pre-β-lipoprotein and α_2-globulin. The so-called pregnancy zone α_2-globulin also appears.

These changes appear to be the result of a direct effect of estrogens on the endoplasmic reticulum of the liver that alters protein production. The clinical implications of many of these changes have not been clearly established.

The changes in the carrier proteins and β-globulin will affect the results of a clinical laboratory test for, *e.g.*, cortisol or thyroid hormones, copper, and iron. An increase in the retinal-binding protein in serum may account for the increased vitamin A serum levels. However, in the presence of a vitamin A deficiency, there may be further tissue depletion of vitamin A.

In animal studies, protein deficiency results in a disease in the endoplasmic reticulum with an increase of glycogen and fat in the liver. In the experimental studies in monkeys noted previously, when hormonal contraceptives were administered there was a significant fall in the levels of serum albumin and total serum proteins in the group of animals on the normal protein diet, whereas changes were not significant in the animals on the low-protein diet (7).

The investigators interpreted these results as possibly indicating that the changes brought on by the low-protein diet alone overshadowed the contraceptive effect. Specific proteins, such as the clotting factors, carrier proteins, etc. were not studied in these experiments.

In this same series of experiments the interaction of hormonal contraceptives, protein deficiency, and liver injury were explored. The effect of a hepatotoxin, aflatoxin, on hemoglobin, albumin, and SGPT were significantly exaggerated by the administration of Ovulen (1 mg ethynodiol diacetate and 0.1 mg mestranol) in protein-deficient animals.

Great care should be exerted in applying the results from controlled animal experiments to human experiences. Because these studies have shown such a potentially deleterious effect from the interaction of malnutrition, endemic diseases resulting in hepatocellular damage, and hormonal contraceptives usage this problem has become a major priority issue in the research program of the World Health Organization.

The epidemiologic association of hormonal contraception and thromboembolic disease has been repeatedly confirmed, although neither the role of clotting factors nor changes in lipid metabolism has been clearly implicated. In the report from the Royal Society of General Practitioners, there was a 5.66-fold increased risk of deep vein thrombosis among oral contraceptive users compared to nonusers (8). The dosage of the estrogen clearly affects this risk, which is decreased but not eliminated at lower dosage levels. At a 50-μg estrogen dose, the rate of superficial vein thrombosis attributable to the hormone would be 30/100,000 women/year.

The role of nutrition and the interaction of nutrition and hormonal contraceptives on thromboembolic disease can only be speculated upon for the present. A comparative study of postoperative thrombosis in the United Kingdom and in Thailand has confirmed the significantly lower incidence of the condition among the Thai women (2). The differences in the clotting factors and fibrinolytic activity noted in some populations in developing countries may be due to racial or nutritional differences. The association of venous thromboembolism with blood group A rather than with group O may explain part of the results in Thailand, since blood group O is found in approximately 80% of Thais. However, several authors have speculated that dietary factors such as the high fat and low residue content of the diet may contribute to the higher incidence of thromboembolic disease, and other disorders, such as obesity and varicose veins, which predispose to thrombophlebitis (1). The question of whether or not hormonal contraceptives increase an already low risk of thromboembolic disease among women in developing countries remains unanswered.

The significance of the increase in α_2-globulins of the renin–angiotensin–aldosterone system is not clearly established despite a well-documented association of oral hormonal contraceptives with hypertension. The role of a nutrition–hormonal contraception interaction on either α_2-globulin changes or hypertension is totally unknown. Levels of plasma renin substrate (PRS), angiotensinogen, and angiotensin II are all found elevated. But they are found to be equally elevated in oral contraceptive users who develop hypertension and those who do not develop hypertension. It has been suggested, but not substantiated, that hypertension (which occurs in up to 15% of women receiving oral contraceptives) may be associated with changes in lipids and carbohydrate metabolism. If the latter is confirmed, a more direct affect of nutrition might exist. Excessive weight gain on oral contraceptives appears to be one of the factors associated with the development of hypertension. The relative risk of developing hypertension while on oral hormones, admittedly affected by a reporting diagnosis bias, was of the order of 2.5 times in the study by the Royal College of General Practitioners (8). The clearest association was that of lower progestogen dose with decreased risk of hypertension. There is no evidence that the dose of estrogen is related to the incidence of hypertension. The risk of hypertension increases with increased duration of use of the preparation. Although only a small percentage of women develop hypertension after prolonged use, both the mean systolic and diastolic pressures are increased from 14 to 8 mm Hg in most users. The relationship of this phenomenon to the development of hypertension in some women is unknown.

The clinical importance of the slight but significant decrease in serum albumin among women on oral hormonal contraceptives is not known. Often, the level of serum albumin is used as an indicator of the adequacy of protein intake. The effect of hormonal contraceptives in the presence of protein deficiency can only be inferred from the very limited animal studies. In the already deficient animal, no further decrease in serum albumin has been noted (7). Such observations must be verified.

LIPID METABOLISM

Hormonal contraceptives have been noted to be associated with increased levels of triglycerides, cholesterol, phospholipids, and lecithin.

The risk of oral contraceptives producing or aggravating occlusive vascular disease in the rare individual with congenital hyperlipidemia has been noted. The significance of the rise in triglycerides and other lipids in normal subjects has not been established, nor has it been established that such changes even take place in women on low-fat diets, such as among women in developing countries.

Elevated serum lipids have been shown to be associated with increased risk of vascular occlusive disease, such as myocardial infarction, in epidemiologic studies. Comparative epidemiologic studies on animal fat in the diet and atherosclerosis have suggested that diet patterns are closely linked to serum lipid levels, and may in turn be linked to the risk of vascular occlusive disease.

Although recent studies on myocardial infarction in reproductive age women show a significant association of oral hormonal contraceptive use and an increased risk of myocardial infarct (4, 5), the available evidence is as yet insufficient to differentiate whether this risk is associated with an increase in coronary artery occlusive disease as might be expected if altered lipid metabolism was the significant change or if an increase in coronary artery thrombosis followed changes in blood clotting factors. In a recently published study the patients with myocardial infarction were noted to have significantly elevated serum cholesterol and triglyceride levels (5). However, in the companion study on myocardial infarct mortality, coronary artery thrombosis was found in 88% of the necropsies of women who died of a myocardial infarct and had been using hormonal contraceptives; whereas, the comparable rate of myocardial deaths in the absence of hormonal contraceptives was 55% (4). The authors note that the necropsies were not done as part of the formal study and that the results may be biased.

The relative risk of hospitalization for a myocardial infarction in a woman using hormonal contraceptives is 2.7/100,000 women/year in the age group 30–39 years and 5.7/100,000 women/year in the group 40–44 years. However, the attributable risk of hospitalization for myocardial infarction was found to be 3.5/100,000 women/year in the age group 30–39 but 47/100,000 women/-year in the group 40–44 years.

WORLD HEALTH ORGANIZATION CONCERN FOR THE PROBLEM

Information on the effects of altered nutrition and hormonal contraceptives has been requested by many governments in the developing world. Several scientific groups and consultative meetings have recommended to WHO that such studies be initiated. In response to these requests the WHO has organized a Task Force on the Interaction of Contraceptive Agents and Methods with Nutritional, Infectious, and Other Health Variables. WHO is currently supporting studies on the interaction of hormonal contraceptives and altered nutrition in three centers in India and Thailand, and studies on the interaction of hormonal contraceptives and schistosomiasis in Egypt. These studies are prospective in design, the women serving as their own controls during 1 year of clinical and laboratory observations.

In addition, studies undertaken by the WHO Research Team on Clinical Evaluation of Fertility Regulating Agents in Bangkok have been related to the interaction of hormonal contraception and nutrition. This group has been responsible for the studies of liver fluke and hormonal contraception, the incidence of thromboembolic disease in Thai women, and DMPA and glucose metabolism.

In the design of these studies, although data are desired on the effect of hormonal contraception on malnutrition or marginal nutrition, the principle of ethical medical practice dictates that women be excluded from the research project if the nutritional status or concurrent disease warrant immediate medical attention. These women are referred to the appropriate health facility for care. Similarly, women who in the course of the study develop certain clinical or laboratory indications of disease or deficiency not originally present, or whose marginal deficiency deteriorates, are not continued in the study but referred to the appropriate health facility for care.

Therefore, built into the design of the prospective studies is a rigid set of inclusion criteria which exclude women with clinically significant nutritional disorders or concurrent disease requiring therapy (Table 14–1).

It was also decided that it would be ethically unacceptable and logistically difficult to select only women with subclinical nutritional deficiencies for the study. It was therefore decided to select communities or population groups as a whole, in which different deficiencies were widely experienced.

Recruitment efforts are made among the entire population in the particular facility or community which meets the criteria for inclusion and to which the investigators have access. A range of variation in nutritional status is expected in such communities, but in addition a clinical and laboratory assessment is carried out in a control population of well-nourished women. Information used in the selection of communities is listed in Table 14–2.

In these and similar studies, the answers to three general questions are being sought as they relate to women with nutritional disorders such as protein, vitamin, or mineral deficiencies if hormonal contraceptives are to be accepted and used with safety, and where such endemic diseases as malaria, schistosomiasis, or tuberculosis exist.

1. Do hormonal contraceptives exacerbate or aggravate an existing borderline deficiency or chronic infection?

Table 14–1. CRITERIA FOR ELIGIBILITY FOR INCLUSION IN WHO-SUPPORTED STUDIES ON THE INTERACTION OF HORMONAL CONTRACEPTION AND NUTRITION

A woman will be eligible for inclusion if she:

(Criteria A—by history)
 1. is between 18 and 35 years of age
 2. is not pregnant
 3. has had no hormonal contraceptives in the last 8 weeks
 4. has no history of renal disease
 5. has no history of jaundice in the last 2 years or jaundice during pregnancy
 6. has no history of hypertension
 7. is not receiving therapy for infections or other diseases*
 8. has aborted more than 6 weeks earlier*
 9. is more than 12 weeks postpartum*
10. is not lactating (unless DMPA accepted) or has been lactating for more than 8 months*
11. has no clinical complaint referable to dietary deficiency

(Criteria B—by physical examination)
 1. has no nutritional edema
 2. has a blood pressure of 140/90 or less
 3. has no clinical evidence of tuberculosis
 4. has no breast masses

(Criteria C—by laboratory examination)
 1. has a hemoglobin level of more than 8.0 g/100 ml
 2. has no evidence of diabetes as measured by the glucose tolerance test

---

*Burkitt, D.P. Br. Med. J. 1:274, 1973

Table 14–2. INFORMATION TO BE USED IN ASSESSING SUITABILITY OF FIELD AREA FOR INTERACTION STUDY

Population
  Total
  Estimates of eligible married women
  Number of women in area receiving contraceptives (from government or private sources)
  Acceptance and discontinuation rates by method

Nutritional status indicators
  Child mortality rates
  Incidence rate of nutritional disorders
  Prevalence of specific nutritional indicators
    Weight for height of school-children
    Skinfold thickness of adult women
    Weight for height of adult women
    Prevalence of anemia in women
  Agricultural production (if rural area)
  Protein consumption patterns

Logistic problems
  Existence of field facility and laboratory
  Time and distance from central laboratory to field area
  Road conditions
  Seasonal variation in accessibility of field area
  Degree of population dispersal
  Number of villages necessary for recruitment of required population
  Number of eligible married women in proposed villages
  Estimate of refusal and drop-out rate among eligible women

2. Are there possible effects of hormonal contraceptives that improve an existing disease state?

3. Is the presence of a nutritional deficiency or other disease associated with a higher or lower risk of the metabolic side effects than have been noted in healthy women?

The implications of the results of research on these questions, if adverse effects are shown, would not necessarily be the rejection of the preparation for use in women with the disease or deficiency condition. If, for example, vitamin deficiency is aggravated, then the strategy of vitamin supplementation possibly would need to be tested. If certain diseases are adversely affected by or affect the metabolic side effects, then treatment regimens should be considered as part of the family planning care or screening systems for women at high risk may have to be developed. Already the supplementation of oral hormonal contraceptives with certain vitamin preparations has been suggested, and in a few instances tested, although not in communities experiencing deficiencies. The alteration of carbohydrate, protein, and lipid metabolism has not been confirmed, nor has the clinical significance been established in populations experiencing nutritional deficiency. Any potential remedial action in terms of altered glucose, protein, or lipid metabolism, if required, would be difficult in communities with limited health resources. Such action might include screening out of individuals at high risk of developing certain complications or the continued monitoring for complications. It is evident that many of the complications are related to the duration of contraceptive use, so that long-term continued unsupervised use might have to be discouraged, and alternative methods of regulating fertility encouraged in certain categories of women. Since the health service requirements for screening, monitoring, and close supervision may be difficult—if not impossible—to mobilize in most developing countries, there is an urgency to confirm the metabolic changes and clinical and epidemiologic implications of any hormonal contraception–nutrition interaction among women in the developing world.

REFERENCES

1. Burkitt DP: Some diseases characteristic of modern western civilization. Br Med J 1:274, 1973
2. Chumnijarakij T, Poshyachinda V: Postoperative thrombosis in Thai women. Lancet 2:1357, 1975
3. Coelingh Bennink HJT, Schreurs WHP: Improvement of oral glucose tolerance in gestational diabetes by pyridoxine. Br Med J 3:13, 1975
4. Mann JI, Inman WHW: Oral contraceptives and death from myocardial infarction. Br Med J 2:245, 1975
5. Mann JI, Vessey MP, Thorogood M, Doll R: Myocardial infarction in young women with special reference to oral contraceptive practice. Br Med J 2:241, 1975
6. Mehrotra ML, Gautam KD, Pande DC, Chaube CK, Dixit R, Malhotra A, Kushwaha S: Compatibility of oral contraceptive with anti-tubercular chemotherapy in female pulmonary tuberculosis patients. Indian J Med Res 62:1782, 1974
7. National Institute of Nutrition, Indian Council of Medical Research, Annual Report. Kanpur, India, 1970, pp 74–79
8. Royal College of General Practitioners: Oral Contraceptives and Health. London, Pitman Medical, 1974
9. Sakr E: Thesis: The effect of contraceptive steroids on bilharzial liver. Cairo, Al Azhar University, 1973
10. Spellacy WN, Buhi WC, Birk SA: The effects of vitamin B_6 on carbohydrate metabolism in women taking steroid contraceptives: preliminary report. Contraception 6:-265, 1972
11. Theuer RC: Effect of oral contraceptive agents on vitamin and mineral needs: a review. J Reprod Med 8:13, 1972
12. WHO: Endocrine Regulation of Human Gestation. (Tech Rep No. 471:5). Geneva, 1971
13. WHO: Advances in Methods of Fertility Regulation. (Tech Rep No. 527:5). Geneva, 1973
14. WHO Research Team on the Clinical Evaluation of Fertility Regulating Agents. Unpublished progress report, 1974
15. WHO: Advances in Methods of Fertility Regulation. (Tech Rep No. 575:5). Geneva, 1975
16. Wynn V: Vitamins and oral contraceptive use. Lancet 1:561, 1975

Chapter 15

Nutrition in Menopausal and Postmenopausal Women

E. Neige Todhunter

The essential role of nutrition in growth and maintenance of the human organism, and the effect of inadequate nutrient intake at all ages have been amply demonstrated in the scientific literature. However, understanding of the role of nutrition during the menopausal period and in the aging process suffers from inadequate experimental evidence and controversial theories. Studies on women, especially after the reproductive period, are limited except for those with clinical conditions. This chapter attempts to bring together and interpret the limited available relevant data concerning the physiology and biochemistry of the menopausal and postmenopausal woman and uses such data as a basis for determining her nutritional requirements.

MENOPAUSE

GENERAL CHARACTERISTICS

Menopause is a stage in the normal progression of women through their total life span. The menopause is the cessation of the menstrual blood flow; it is preceded by menstrual irregularities and is followed by physiologic changes and adjustments to changes in ovarian function. This total is the *climacteric,* more frequently referred to as *menopause* or the menopausal period.

Menopause occurs generally between 45 and 50 years of age but may occur anytime between 35 and 60 years (87). Authorities ascribe slightly different ages to this period, such as 45 to 48 years (59), about 50 years (13, 55), and 49 years (77). Menopause is the visible evidence of atrophic changes in the ovaries and diminution in estrogen production. The physiologic changes with menopause are common to all women, but there is wide variation in the extent and intensity of overt symptoms, ranging from none to severe. It is estimated that only 15–25% of menopausal women experience sufficient discomfort and problems to send them to a physician (55, 77, 87). Many of the myths and stereotypes about menopause are disappearing as women move from home to the career world and become more knowledgeable about their own physiology and the freedoms available to them in the sixth decade and later years of life (52).

SYMPTOMS AT MENOPAUSE

These are grouped as: a) Symptoms related to the autonomic nervous system, including hot flushes of the head, neck, and upper part of the thorax accompanied by excessive perspiration and hot flashes which may involve the whole body (31, 55). Also there may be gastrointestinal complaints and numbness and tingling in fingers. b) Psychosomatic disturbances including headaches, irritability, depression, personality changes, and nervousness accompanied by loss of appetite or compulsive eating. These changes are dependent on the state of health, emotional maturity, and stability when entering the menopausal period and may not be caused primarily by menopause (59). c) Somatic changes which include alterations in the reproductive tract, the musculoskeletal system, and endocrine system (31).

ENDOCRINE CHANGES

The fine balance of endocrine secretions, which is an essential part of the normal reproductive period, is no longer maintained when the female enters the menopausal period. With ovarian failure, there is a decrease in estrogen production and a reciprocal rise in the secretion of follicle-stimulating hormone (FSH) and luteinizing hormone (LH) from the pituitary (1, 87).

Parathyroid hormone levels in serum of women aged 65 and over are significantly higher than those in young women age 20 (7). All hormones appear to play some part in the regulation of cellular metabolism and control of physiologic responses. Since many of the hormones have an inhibiting or stimulating effect on each other, it can be reasoned that these and other hormonal changes will influence metabolic changes and nutrient requirements of older women (24, 40, 93).

BIOLOGIC CHANGES IN WOMEN AFTER FORTY

GENERAL COMMENTS

Biologic changes will affect nutritional processes and nutrient requirements. Extensive reports are available on aging changes in man, some from longitudinal studies (6, 32, 72), but most from cross-sectional studies of males. Comparatively few data are available for women and none except endocrine changes for the menopausal woman. Since menopause is a physiologic incident in the life of every woman, endocrine changes are directly associated with this age period. Other changes have not yet been identified as related to menopause.

Aging changes proceed at diverse rates in individuals, and various organs are affected differently (72). In general, the aging changes reported for man (and assumed to follow the same trends in women) are decreasing cardiac output, especially after age 40; a decrease of about 20% between ages 30 and 90 in basal metabolic rate (based on surface area calculations); declining renal blood flow after age 35 to 40; decreased glomerular filtration rate of about 0.6%/year after age 30, ascribed to loss of functioning nephrons; decreased vital capacity and maximal breathing capacity; and impairment of some cellular functions such as reduction in activity of some enzymes (32, 72). Decline in total body water, with the greater loss being in the intracellular compartment, has also been reported (39); bone loss also occurs (25, 29).

BODY COMPOSITION

The female body composition and the extent and rate of changes differ from that of the male (84). Young and coworkers (90, 91, 92) have attempted to provide normative data on body fatness of 94 normal women—as a basis for studying changes with age—using newer techniques of densitometry and total body water determination from which body fatness can be determined. These and other measurements for young women 16 to 30 years age were used as a basis of comparison for women 30 to 70 years of age. Measurements of the older age group were expressed as percent change from the base data on younger women. Mean body weight increased with the fifth decade and remained high. Mean body density decreased at the fifth decade and hence body fatness increased after the fortieth year; increases were 23.1% at 40–50 years, 46.0% at 50–60 years, and 55.3% at 60–70 years. Skinfold thickness showed little change until 40 years of age, when it increased 22.1%. It increased only slightly thereafter, indicating no further deposition of fat in subcutaneous tissues. Additional evidence that fat deposition was abdominal was obtained from soft tissue x-rays and circumference measurements of parts of the body. Basal oxygen consumption per kilogram body weight and total body water as percent of body weight decreased slightly but consistently each decade; the creatinine coefficient also decreased but less consistently. Residual air in the lungs increased with each decade (91).

Other investigators found the percent of body fat increased in women from 25–55 years and then decreased (10); the fat content of women, mean age 39, was 23% (29), and the increase in fat was in the abdominal area (73).

BLOOD CONSTITUENTS

Blood levels of nutrients and metabolic products are one of the useful indicators of nutritional status and physiologic changes. Normal values are essential as a base line for determination of significant differences, but few such data are available for women covering the age range of maturity to old age. Values for some blood constituents are dependent on sex and age, and some directly reflect dietary intake. More sophisticated equipment and techniques now provide some statistically significant data on this (2, 57, 63, 68, 87).

Aging Effect

Blood volume, pH, red cell count, and osmotic pressure show little if any change with age (72). In both men and women there is a decrease with age in the levels of calcium, phosphorus, total protein, and albumin, and an increase in levels of glucose, urea nitrogen, cholesterol, and lactic dehydrogenase. With age, uric acid increases in women (57).

Sex Difference

Iron has long been recognized as present in lower levels in women. Calcium, glucose, urea nitrogen, and uric acid levels are significantly higher in men than in women (57). Significant differences have also been found between the sexes in levels of alkaline phosphatase, creatinine, total protein, and albumin (68).

Menopause

Wilding *et al.* (88) report significant increases in eight blood constituents in women between the fifth and sixth decades, when physiologic changes associated with estrogen insufficiency are also occurring. These serum constituents are urea, uric acid, inorganic phosphate, calcium, alkaline phosphatase, cholesterol, total lipids, and sodium. Also, estrogen levels decrease at menopause, but Wilding *et al.* (88) propose that the physiologic changes at this period are much too complex for all of them to be explained by changes in estrogen secretion. He raises the question whether different blood data may be obtained when analyses are made on a new generation of menopausal women who have taken contraceptive pills (88). Serum parathyroid hormone levels are markedly increased by some tenfold in women between the ages of 20 and 65 years (7).

Dietary Effects

With age, blood levels for calcium, iron, trace elements, lipids, and cholesterol change in women and will be discussed below, as will several of the vitamins since blood levels of these are susceptible to dietary influences.

CLINICAL CONDITIONS WITH NUTRITION-RELATED FACTORS

THE OVERWEIGHT INDIVIDUAL

Weight of 10–20% in excess of normal weight for height at age 25 and in relation to body composition or body build is considered *overweight*. Individual variations in body build make it difficult to assess the "normal" or desirable weight, and there is no agreement as to how much should be considered excess. *Obesity* is excessive accumulation of fat; this can be determined by skinfold measures and body density determinations. Weight 30% above desirable is considered to be obesity (44). The basic cause is intake of calories greater than energy expenditure; there is a higher incidence of obesity among women than men. Hormonal changes may be a factor, but knowledge of this is limited apart from the effect of thyroid activity. Some middle-aged and many older women tend to decrease their physical activity but maintain their accustomed dietary patterns and caloric intake. Food intake may be used as compensation for tension and frustration, and other psychologic factors may be involved. The clinical hazards of obesity are recognized (44).

DIABETES MELLITUS

There appears to be no sex difference in diabetes prevalence for persons under age 40; at ages 40 and over the rates for females are substantially higher (45). Many different factors can produce diabetes or increase the risk of the disease, the most important being obesity and genetic factors (85). Whether menopausal changes are a factor is not clear. According to West (85), the factor most strongly and consistently associated with prevalence of adult-onset diabetes is the degree and duration of adiposity and the most important dietary factor is total calorie intake, irrespective of source. Currently there is decreasing emphasis on the priority formerly given to carbohydrate restriction. Emphasis is on diets for diabetics that are lower in saturated fat and cholesterol than the previous traditional regimens because of the increasing vulnerability of postmenopausal women to coronary disease and the high rate of this disease in diabetics (85).

CORONARY HEART DISEASE AND ATHEROSCLEROSIS

Coronary heart disease (CHD) is a major cause of death in this country. Studies of mortality rates from CHD show that white females have a lower death rate than males. The death rate for females increases steadily with age, but slows down for males at about age 45. Nonwhite females have a substantially higher death rate than white females at each age grouping up to 65 years. The mortality data do not support the hypothesis that estrogenic activity affords premenopausal females relative protection against death from CHD. There is no change in rate of increase of death rates following the age of menopause (49).

Atherosclerosis is recognized as a major underlying cause of CHD (19, 49, 76), and there is strong evidence that nutrition and metabolism are centrally involved (49). Statistical analyses of data obtained from the International Atherosclerosis Project have shown significant correlations between atherosclerotic lesions and serum cholesterol levels, and percent of calories from fat. Correlations between lesions and percent of animal fat in total dietary fat and sugar composition were not significant (76). Atherosclerotic lesions were increased in persons with hypertension and diabetes (76).

Beneficial results in control of atherogenesis have been reported from diets of limited fat and cholesterol intake (89). Atherosclerosis and CHD are multifactorial in etiology (49), but there is considerable agreement that diet lowers serum cholesterol and triglyceride levels and significantly reduces atherosclerosis and new clinical coronary artery disease events (44, 67, 76, 89). Current dietary recommendations include 1) controlled caloric intake to prevent obesity, 2) amount and type of fat controlled to prevent hyperlipidemia, 3) use of complex rather than refined carbohydrates, and 4) limited salt intake to prevent any tendency to hypertension (5).

A recent hypothesis (41) is that the ratio of zinc to copper may be the preponderant factor in etiology of coronary heart disease. A relative or absolute deficiency of copper causes this high ratio, resulting in hypercholesterolemia and increased CHD mortality. Further investigation is needed.

OSTEOPOROSIS

Osteoporosis is a commonly appearing disorder among women especially after menopause, probably beginning around age 35–45 in women and about 45–65 years in men (3). Estimates of the incidence vary, but is reported to occur in at least 1 of 4 postmenopausal women (71).

This disease is characterized by reduced bone tissue relative to the volume of anatomic bone; so far as known the chemical composition remains normal (54). There is increased bone resorption in the osteoporotic patient. The literature on osteoporosis is extensive, and the theories are numerous but without agreement on causative factors or treatment (28, 74). Problems include the measurement of bone density, the extreme difficulty of fully controlled studies on humans, the difficulty in obtaining reference standards for what is normal bone and osteoporotic bone, and the development of accurate and reproducible methods for repetitive measures of bone mass (28).

Low calcium content of the diet may be a factor, but the effects of increased calcium intake or calcium supplements are contradictory (54, 86). Prevalence of reduced bone density was found to be higher in women in towns in North Dakota where the fluoride content of soil and water was low, compared with those in communities with high levels of fluoride in the same state (8). Treatment of osteoporotic subjects with fluoride has not produced positive results; possibly, the fluoride is most effective in the bone structure before maturity. Other factors considered important in preventing the bone fragility associated with osteoporosis are endocrine changes at menopause, decreased activity or immobilization, loss of muscle tone, normal aging processes, and other nutritional factors such as phosphate, vitamin D, and acid–base balance (60, 86).

Much more research is necessary to clarify this problem in menopausal and older women even though there is fair agreement that diet is a factor involved. Albanese *et al.* (3) believe it is clear that osteoporosis has a nutrition component but that this component is not solely a calcium deficiency.

NUTRIENT REQUIREMENTS AND AGING

INFLUENCING FACTORS

A daily dietary intake of all nutrients is essential for individuals of all ages and stages of the life cycle, but the amount of each nutrient required is influenced by a number of factors. The preceding discussion has presented some evidence that there are physiologic changes associated with the aging process and with menopause distinct from aging. These and other data suggest that the following factors influence the quantitative nutrient requirements of menopausal and older women: 1) nutritional status at the times of menopause, 2) body weight and body composition, 3) endocrine changes, 4) physical activity, 5) metabolic changes, 6) functional disorders, and 7) muscular efficiency and basal metabolic rate which tend to decrease with age.

RECOMMENDED DIETARY ALLOWANCES

Nutritional requirements for women have received little investigative attention except during pregnancy and lactation. The Food and Nutrition Board of the National Research Council first formulated tables of Recommended Dietary Allowances (RDA) in 1943. These have been revised periodically in the light of new data; the most recent revision was published in 1974 (18). The RDA are not requirements; they are estimates only for energy and for 17 nutrients. The allowances are intended to be adequate to meet nutritional needs of practically all healthy persons. They are based on available scientific knowledge; therefore, the menopausal woman receives no attention, nor is her age period or that of the middle-aged woman given any consideration. Age groupings for the adult female are 23–50 and 51+ years.

The RDAs serve as the available guide to dietary allowances for women. Similar types of tables, but with different quantitative allowances, have been prepared in many other countries, and the Food and Agriculture Organization (FAO) in cooperation with the World Health Organization agencies of the United Nations have prepared international tables (33). Recommended intakes are given only for an adult woman, moderately active. Individual intakes below recommended levels are not necessarily indicative of deficiency.

PROTEINS AND AMINO ACIDS

The RDA for any female over 22 years of age is 46, and FAO recommendation is 37 g (18, 33).

Balance studies on older women are contradictory; some find an increased and some a lower requirement for protein for older women compared with young sedentary women; others indicate that it is similar (36, 37). Difference in protein quality, the amino acid composition, is well recognized (4). Recommended intakes of protein are on the assumption that the diet has sufficient animal sources of protein to compensate for amino acid deficiencies or imbalances in plant proteins. Requirement of the essential amino acids, those that must be supplied in the performed state in the diet, have been established for college-age women but not for older women (36, 37, 50). The quantitative requirement for essential amino acids declines with age, and the major requirement appears to be for adequate amino nitrogen in the adult (50).

FATS AND FATTY ACIDS

The RDA makes no quantitative recommendation for fat intake at any age. Fat is an important source of calories and contributes to the palatability and satiety values of the diet. Dietary fat is a source of essential fatty acids and fat-soluble vitamins. The essential fatty acids, linoleic acid and arachidonic acid, are polyunsaturated. Linoleic acid can be converted to arachidonic acid and is found in high concentration in many vegetable oils but not in coconut or olive oil (18).

The essential fatty acids have a role in cholesterol transport and metabolism.

Diets high in the polyunsaturates have been shown to reduce the serum levels of cholesterol in man, though there is also contradictory evidence. Essential fatty acids are structural components of phospholipids and are precursors of prostaglandins (18).

The required intake of essential fatty acids is between 1–2% of the total calories, and this level is readily achieved in the ordinary diet (18).

CARBOHYDRATE AND ENERGY REQUIREMENTS

Little attention has been paid to carbohydrates and aging. The carbohydrates are a major source of calories, and the highly refined carbohydrate has been implicated as a possible atherogenic factor (83). Carbohydrate plays a metabolic role in the prevention of ketosis, excessive breakdown of body protein, loss of cations (especially sodium), and involuntary dehydration (18). There is no quantitative requirement for carbohydrate. Common dietary practice is to obtain 45–65% of the total calories from carbohydrate. Dietary control of carbohydrate is important in diabetes mellitus, which has a high incidence in older women.

Energy requirements are assessed in kilocalories or kilojoules (1 kcal is equivalent to 4.184 kJ). The RDA for females aged 23–50 is 2000 kcal, but individual requirements vary widely, body size and activity being the determining factors. Reduction of caloric intake with increasing age requires greater care in food selection so that the nutrient intakes are not decreased.

FAT-SOLUBLE VITAMINS

Vitamin A

This is the generic term for biologically active compounds showing vitamin A activity: retinol (vitamin A_1) and its esters; retinal; retinoic acid; and carotenoids with provitamin A activity. Vitamin A activity, formerly expressed in international units (IU), is now measured in retinol equivalents (RE). One RE is equal to 3.33 IU of retinol or 10 IU of β-carotene (18).

The RDA for women over 23 years of age is 800 μg RE, and the FAO recommendation for a moderately active woman is 750 μg. Vitamin A absorption is unchanged by aging (83), and women who regularly consume green and yellow vegetables should have no difficulty in meeting vitamin A requirements.

Vitamin D

There is no RDA for women, but FAO recommends 2.5 μg as cholecalciferol which is vitamin D_3. This vitamin is converted to 25-hydroxycholecalciferol in the liver and to 1,25-dihydroxycholecalciferol in the kidney (9, 21). Inadequate intakes of vitamin D or disorders interfering with the absorption of vitamin D, calcium, and phosphorus may lead to senile osteomalacia (83). Older women without access to sunshine may be low in vitamin D. Excessive intakes of vitamin D are toxic.

Vitamin E

No evidence of vitamin E deficit is available for adults nor is there clarification of its function in human metabolism. The vitamin E activity available in the average American diet is considered satisfactory, and the RDA for adult females is 12 IU (18).

WATER-SOLUBLE VITAMINS

Thiamine and Riboflavin

Thiamine is required at all ages. There is some evidence that older persons use thiamine less efficiently. The RDA for all adult women is 1 mg/day, and this intake should be maintained even on low-calorie diets (18). FAO recommends 0.9 mg/day for adult women (33).

Riboflavin is widely distributed in foods, and there is some evidence of deficiency in the average diet. The RDA for women over 50 years is 1.1 mg/day, and FAO recommends 1.3 mg for adult women.

Vitamin B_6

This is the collective term for pyridoxine, pyridoxal, and pyridoxamine, which are interconvertible *in vivo*. There is interaction of vitamin B_6 with steroid hormones. The use of oral steroid contraceptives is accompanied by increased excretion of tryptophan metabolites following a tryptophan load, and a variety of symptoms of malaise and increased amounts of pyridoxine are required to correct these conditions (18). Evidence is not available regarding vitamin B_6 requirement for women at menopause or those receiving estrogen therapy at this period.

There is some evidence that vitamin B_6 requirements increase with age (38) and with high-protein diets (14). Dietary deprivation of vitamin B_6 has been reported to lead to depression and confusion in adults (18). The RDA for women over 23 years age is 2.0 mg/day.

Niacin

Niacin is the generic term for nicotinic acid and nicotinamide, and is concerned with glycolysis, fat synthesis, and tissue respiration. Tryptophan can be converted to niacin; a dietary intake of 60 mg of tryptophan provides about 1 mg niacin. The classic deficiency disease pellagra occurs in patients on diets high in maize because of a deficiency of niacin and of proteins containing tryptophan.

The RDA for niacin for women age 23–50 is 13 mg/day and for women over 50 years is 12 mg/day (18). FAO recommends 14.5 mg/day for adult women (33).

Vitamin B_{12}

Vitamin B_{12}, cyanocobalamin, is a component of several coenzymes concerned with nucleic acid formation. Deficiency is characterized by megaloblastic anemia. Vitamin B_{12} is present only in animal foodstuffs and requires an intrinsic factor, a glycoprotein, for its absorption from the intestinal tract. The RDA for adult women is 3.0 mg/day. FAO recommends 2.0 mg/day.

Folacin

Folacin is the generic term for folic acid (pteroylglutamic acid) and related compounds that exhibit the biologic activity of folic acid. This vitamin is present in a wide variety of foods, but there is considerable loss in food preparation and some concern that diets may be low in folacin. The RDA recommendation for adult women is 400 µg/day. FAO recommendation is 200 µg/day.

Drugs commonly prescribed in old age may interfere with folic acid metabolism (30).

Ascorbic Acid

Ascorbic acid, vitamin C, is traditionally associated with scurvy. It functions in the synthesis of collagen, the metabolic reactions of amino acids, and the synthesis of epinephrine and antiinflammatory steroids by the adrenal gland, and is associated with impaired wound healing (18). No increased requirement has been reported in the elderly, but conditions of stress and drug therapy may increase the need for this vitamin. The requirement for the adult female is assumed to be the same as for the adult male, 45 mg/day for women over 23 years of age. FAO recommends 30 mg/day for the adult women. For those women who do not have a daily intake of fruits and vegetables, deficiency of ascorbic acid is possible.

MINERALS

Calcium

The body calcium of a 70-kg adult is approximately 1200 g, with 99% present in the skeleton. The remaining calcium outside of bone is in extracellular fluids and soft tissues where its role is in controlling excitability of peripheral nerves and muscle. Calcium functions in blood coagulation, myocardial action, muscle contractility, and maintenance of the integrity of various membranes (18) and possibly in as yet unknown biochemical systems (3). In controlled studies of elderly females, calcium has been reported to have a hypocholesterolemic effect (3).

The desirable intake of calcium to maintain these functions is a subject of disagreement. The RDA is 800 mg for women after 23 years of age and is based largely on calcium balance experiments (18). FAO recommended intake for adult women is 400–500 mg. This difference in recommendation reflects the disagreement between investigators. There are those who believe that humans adapt to comparatively low intakes of calcium such as seen in many underdeveloped countries where there is no evidence of calcium deficiency. Others interpret the evidence to show benefits when calcium intakes are of the order of 800 mg or more (17, 18).

Calcium absorption is around 30% of the intake. Factors which influence absorption are vitamin D intake; the dietary presence of oxalates and phytic acid (though these are not significant unless the calcium intake is low); and a calcium to phosphorus ratio between 2:1 and 1:2, though wide variation is tolerated if vitamin D is adequate (18). Calcium metabolism is influenced by protein intake; urinary calcium excretion is markedly increased when the calcium intake is held constant and the protein intake increased (16).

The problems of calcium metabolism and calcium requirement are as yet unresolved, and further research is necessary on the requirements of the menopausal woman and the physiologic stresses she undergoes, including emotional stress. Earlier studies (56) with adolescent girls and mature adults have shown that positive calcium balances became negative under emotional stress and reverted to positive balances when the tension was relieved.

Phosphorus

The phosphorus allowance for women is similar to that for calcium, 800 mg/day (18). Phosphorus combines with calcium to form bone. It is also present in blood cells, lipids, proteins, and carbohydrates and in energy transfer enzymes. Combination with phosphate in the body is essential before many of the B vitamins can function (18). It is widely distributed in foods, and a dietary deficiency has not been observed in humans.

Iron

The menopausal woman is relieved of the loss of iron in the menstrual flow which varies widely but may be as high as 1.5 mg/day. She still requires iron for its normal functions as a constituent of hemoglobin, myoglobin, and a number of enzymes. The RDA for women over 50 years age is 10 mg/day (18, 64).

The body has no physiologic mechanism for excretion of absorbed iron. Iron equilibrium is maintained largely by regulation of the amount of iron absorbed. Absorption from food by healthy subjects is between 5% and 10% of the ingested amount, while iron-deficient subjects absorb 10–20% or more. Iron absorption is controlled by the intestinal mucosa, the amount and chemical nature of the iron in the food ingested, other dietary factors which increase or decrease the availability of iron for absorption, and by the state of body reserves of iron (65). Controlled studies using biosynthetically labeled foodstuffs fed as a single food show the mean absorption of iron from vegetable foods to range from 1% for rice and spinach to 6% from soybeans. Absorption from animal foods ranged from 7% for ferritin to 22% from veal muscle. Other foods added to the single test food caused change in the iron absorption. Meat increased the amount absorbed from foods such as maize or blackbeans; cysteine was one substance responsible for this enhancing effect. Vitamin C increased the absorption from nonheme food iron, while egg and phytates decreased it. In a mixed diet of the type eaten in this country, iron absorption was 6% in iron-deficient subjects (65). Iron deficiency anemia results in lowered hemoglobin, plasma iron below 40 μg/100 ml, an elevated iron-binding capacity, and less than 15% saturation of the transferrin. Excessive intakes and high absorption of iron can lead to an iron overload and excessive storage as hemosiderin. Danger of such an occurrence for the menopausal woman seems negligible; her problem and that of older women is the selection of a diet adequate in iron.

Iodine

Iodine is essential for the formation of the thyroid hormones thyroxine (T_4) and triiodothyronine (T_3). Inadequate intakes of iodine lead to endemic or simple goiter as evidenced by enlargement of the gland. Some factors not yet clearly identified may be causative in some endemic areas, and goitrogens have been found in some foods such as the cabbage family. Iodine content of foods is dependent on the soil, and in many areas of the United States where iodine has been leached from the soil, the use of iodized salt is recommended. The RDA for iodine is 100 μg for females age 23–50 years and 80 μg after age 50 (18).

Magnesium

Magnesium, next to potassium, is the predominant cation in living cells and is an essential part of many enzyme systems (18). It has a fundamental role in most reactions that include phosphate transfer and probably is essential in the structural stabilization of nucleic acids. Severe deficiency impairs the homeostasis of both potassium and calcium and may lead to neuromuscular dysfunction (66). Deficiency may occur in children and be a complication of kwashiorkor but is infrequent in adults except alcoholics.

Magnesium is widely distributed in plant foods; meat is also a rich source. The RDA for adult females is 300 mg.

Newly Identified Trace Elements

The trace elements required for human nutrition are only now being identified when sophisticated instruments and methodology become available to detect their presence in biologic materials at levels of parts per million or, in some cases, parts per billion. Many of these mineral elements function in enzyme systems, and future research could possibly show their significance for older women. These trace elements appear to be widely distributed in food (66).

Zinc, chromium, copper, molybdenum, manganese, cobalt, selenium, and fluoride are all believed to be essential in human nutrition, and vanadium, tin, silicon, and nickel have been identified as required by some animals and possibly are essential for man (48).

Zinc Considerable data are now available on zinc (61). Growth failure, sexual infantilism in teenage individuals, idiopathic hypogeusia, and impaired wound healing appear in man as a result of zinc deficiency (22). Decreased protein synthesis associated with depressed activity of RNA and DNA polymerases is observed in zinc-deficient plants and animals (61). Most of the body zinc is in the bones, with an approximate concentration of 200 μg/g; muscles contain about 50 μg/g and plasma concentrations range from 80–110 μg/g (66). Excretion is mainly by way of the feces. Zinc is widely distributed in foods, but the availability may be reduced by phytates which bind zinc particularly in the presence of calcium (51). The RDA for zinc for females over 23 years of age is 15 mg/day.

Copper Copper is essential in the utilization of iron. It has a function in the maintenance of myelin and is a component of several amine oxidases and other enzymes, and of ceruloplasmin and some other copper-containing proteins (18, 35, 66). Copper, like zinc, helps to maintain normal taste sensitivity (30). Liver, fish, and green vegetables are usually good sources of copper, containing over 100 μg/100 kcal; relatively poor sources with less than 50 μg/100 kcal are milk, cheese, beef, bread, and breakfast cereals. WHO suggests an intake of 30 μg/kg per day for adult males but makes no reference to females (66).

Chromium Trivalent chromium plays a part in glucose metabolism. Insulin-requiring diabetics show abnormalities in chromium metabolism and impaired glucose tolerance (66). It also has a function in nucleic acid metabolism (46, 47). Low levels of chromium are found in the tissues of older subjects. Requirements have not yet been quantified.

Molybdenum Molybdenum has been identified in xanthine oxidase and several other enzymes and is required by man. No recommended daily allowance has been established.

Manganese Manganese is required by man but no deficiency symptoms have been observed. It is part of enzyme systems of man (18). No recommended daily allowance has been established.

Cobalt Cobalt is classified with the essential trace elements because it is physiologically active in man in the form of vitamin B_{12}, cyanocobalamin, and adequate intakes of this vitamin are essential (18, 66).

Selenium Selenium is considered essential for man and may influence the synthesis of glutathione and protein. It appears to enhance the absorption of α-tocopherol and so reduce the requirement for vitamin E (70). Deficiency symptoms have not been observed, and the quantitative requirement is not known (43).

Fluorine Fluorine functions in tooth structure in maximal resistance to dental caries during infancy and childhood, an effect which persists through adult life.

Fluorine also is incorporated into bone structure and may be effective in resistance to osteoporosis.

Fluorine and all of the trace elements are toxic when consumed in excessive amounts (69).

Other Trace Elements Other trace elements—silicon, nickel, tin, and vanadium —have been shown to be essential for the rat and/or the chick, but nothing is yet known about them in human nutrition (15, 53).

WATER

Water is an essential nutrient for daily replacement of the body water component. The normal rate of turnover in adults is about 6% of the total body water content. A liberal intake of water may aid in improving elimination (83); very high protein diets lead to increased water requirement. With a decreased basal metabolic rate, less water is required, but there is no data on water needs of older people. Many factors influence body water loss, and the requirement is only an estimate. There is no RDA for water intake, but a reasonable allowance is given as 1 mg/kcal for adults (18).

DIETARY FIBER

Fiber of plants consists of lignin, cellulose, and hemicellular and pectin materials, with content varying with the type of plant and its structure (80). Currently, research has indicated a possible relation between fiber and the bulk and transit time of stools through the colon (11, 12, 58) and also with diseases of the gastrointestinal tract and lowering of plasma lipids (23, 82). These effects need to be clarified by further research, and any dietary fiber or fiber constituent identified. Whatever the outcome of further study, increasing the natural fiber content of the average diet today has merit. Beneficial effects in preventing constipation are recognized, and vegetables, fruits, and less-refined cereal products have the advantage of increasing the intake of vitamins (especially vitamin C in fruits and vegetables) and minerals, particularly trace elements.

NUTRITIONAL STATUS AND DIETARY SURVEYS

How does the menopausal and older woman fare when her nutritional status and dietary adequacy is studied? The menopausal woman has not been specifically studied, but there have been studies of the middle aged and those over age 60.

Biochemical determinations of nutrient-related constituents of blood and urine are one measure of nutritional status. Such data should be interpreted with caution because of lack of agreement regarding the basis of acceptable or normal levels. Also, there is wide variation in acceptable levels among normal healthy individuals. Biochemical data show population and aging trends and help to identify groups which may be at risk of developing physiologic or metabolic disturbances related to nutrient deficiencies.

The recent Ten-State Survey (78) provides biochemical data by sex, age, and ethnic groups for some nutrient-related constituents of blood and urine. Females were grouped by ages 35–59 years and 60 years and over. Biochemical values were usually related to income level. There was a comparatively small percentage receiving low or deficient ratings for protein and the vitamins. Dietary data were obtained from 24-hour recall (79). Calorie intakes were low for women over 66, therefore, they often failed to meet the nutrient standards for their age and weight. Limiting nutrients were protein, iron, and vitamin A; black women had poorer diets than white women. Dietary intakes were closely related to biochemical findings. Women had lower intakes than males for all nutrients except vitamin C. The data for women over 60 were comparable to those obtained in the U.S. Department of Agriculture dietary survey of 1965 (26).

The recent preliminary report (62) of the 1971–1972 Health and Nutrition Examination Survey (Hanes) has not yet provided data on women in the middle and older age groups.

Other dietary studies have been on a more localized basis for women over 60 years age (20, 27, 34, 42, 75, 81). Nutrients most frequently at levels below recommended intakes were thiamine, iron, and calcium. Dietary intakes decreased with age, income, and educational level. Some groups frequently took vitamin and mineral supplements.

GENERAL CONCLUSIONS

There is no evidence that nutrient requirements are increased or decreased by menopausal changes, except for a decrease in iron requirement. It is of first importance for women to enter the middle years in good nutritional status and in good physical condition to meet the possible stress of endocrine changes at menopause and the physiologic changes that occur in the aging process with its accompanying hazards of osteoporosis, diabetes, cardiovascular disease, and obesity.

With increasing years, when physical activity lessens, the energy intake should be decreased while the nutrient intake remains the same. Meals that provide a variety of foods offer the best means of meeting the nutrient needs. When clinical treatment requires dietary modifications and the food prescription cannot provide all essentials, then nutrient supplements must be provided.

More research is needed on the physiologic changes in adult females to establish normal baselines for body composition, blood constituents, and functional changes and to determine quantitative requirements for women of all ages, especially at menopause and in the later years of life.

REFERENCES

1. Adamopoulus DA, Loraine JA, Dove GA: Endocrinological studies in women approaching the menopause. J Obstet Gynaecol Br Commonw 78:62, 1971
2. Adlersberg D, Schaefer LE, Steinberg AG, Wang CI: Age, sex, serum lipids and coronary atherosclerosis. JAMA 162:619, 1956
3. Albanese AA, Edelson AH, Woodhull ML, Lorenze EJ Jr, Wein EH, Orto LA: Effect of a calcium supplement on serum cholesterol, calcium, phosphorus, and bone density of "normal healthy" elderly females. Nutr Rep Int 8:119, 1973
4. Albanese AA, Orto LA: The proteins and amino acids. In Goodhart RS, Shils ME (eds): Modern Nutrition in Health and Disease, 5th ed. Philadelphia, Lea & Febiger, 1973, pp 28–88
5. American Health Foundation: Position statement on diet and coronary heart disease. Developed by Christakis G, Rathman D: Prev Med 1:255, 1972
6. Baker SP, Shock NW, Norris AH: Basal metabolism and body water in women. In Shock NW (ed): Biological Aspects of Aging. New York, Columbia University Press, 1962, pp 88–89
7. Berlyne GM, Ben–Ari J, Galinsky D, Hirsch M, Kushelevesky A, Shainkin R: The etiology of osteoporosis; the role of parathyroid hormone. JAMA 229:1904, 1974
8. Bernstein DS, Sadowsky N, Hegsted DM, Guri CD, Stare FJ: Prevalence of osteoporosis in high- and low-fluoride areas in North Dakota. JAMA 198:499, 1966
9. Bordier P, Pechet MM, Hesse R, Rasmussen PM, Rasmussen H: Response of adult patients with osteomalacia to treatment with crystalline 1α-hydroxy vitamin D_3. N Engl J Med 291:866, 1974
10. Brozek J, Chen KP, Carlton W, Bronczyk F: Age and sex difference in man's fat content during maturity (abstr). Fed Proc 12:21, 1953
11. Burkitt DP: Epidemiology of large bowel disease: the role of fibre. Proc Nutr Soc 32:145, 1973
12. Burkitt DP, Walker ARP, Painter NS: Effect of dietary fibre on stools and transmit-times and its role in the causation of disease. Lancet 2:1408, 1972
13. Cali RW: Management of the climacteric and menopausal woman. Med Clin North Am 56:789, 1972
14. Canham JE, Baker EM, Harding RS, Sauberlich HE, Plough IC: Dietary protein—its relationship to Vitamin B_6 requirements and function. Ann NY Acad Sci 166:16, 1969
15. Carlisle EM: Silicon as an essential element. Fed Proc 33:1758, 1974
16. Chu JY, Margen S, Costa FM: Studies in calcium metabolism. II. Effects of low calcium and variable protein intake on human calcium metabolism. Am J Clin Nutr 28:1028, 1975
17. Cohn SH, Dombrowski CS, Hauser W, Atkins HL: High calcium diet and the parameters of calcium metabolism in osteoporosis. Am J Clin Nutr 21:1246, 1968
18. Committee on Dietary Allowances: Recommended dietary allowances, 8th revised ed. Washington DC, Food and Nutrition Board, National Research Council, National Academy of Sciences, 1974
19. Connor WE, Connor SL: The key role of nutritional factors in the prevention of coronary heart disease. Prev Med 1:49, 1972
20. Davidson CS, Livermore J, Anderson P, Kaufman S: The nutrition of a group of apparently healthy aging persons. Am J Clin Nutr 10:181, 1962
21. DeLuca HF: Recent advances in the metabolism and function of Vitamin D. Fed Proc 28: 1678, 1969
22. Editorial: Zinc in human medicine. Lancet 2:351, 1975
23. Editorial: Dietary fibre and plasma-lipids. Lancet 2:353, 1975
24. Eisenstein AB, Singh SP: Hormonal control of nutrient metabolism. In Goodhart RS, Shils ME (eds): Modern Nutrition in Health and Disease, 5th ed. Philadelphia, Lea & Febiger, 1973, pp 457–473

25. Exton–Smith AN: Physiological aspects of aging: relationship to nutrition. Am J Clin Nutr 25:853, 1972
26. Food intake and nutritive value of diets of men, women and children in the United States, Spring 1965, a preliminary report. Washington DC, Agricultural Research Service, US Department of Agriculture, ARS–62–18, March, 1969
27. Fry PC, Fox HM, Linkswiler H: Nutrient intakes of healthy older women. J Am Diet Assoc 42:218, 1963
28. Gallagher JC, Nordin BEC: Calcium metabolism and the menopause. In Curry AS, Hewitt JV (eds): Biochemistry of Women: Clinical Concepts. Cleveland, CRC Press, 1974, pp 145–163
29. Garn SM: Fat weight and fat placement in the female. Science 125:1091, 1957
30. Girdwood RH: Deficiencies of folic acid and vitamin B_{12}. In Exton–Smith AN, Scott DL (eds): Vitamins in the Elderly. London, J Wright & Sons, 1968, p 40
31. Goldfarb AF: Menopause, the climacteric: its role in aging. Med Sci 18:48, 1967
32. Goldman R: Decline in organ function with aging. In Rossman I (ed): Clinical Geriatrics. Philadelphia, JB Lippincott, 1971, pp 20–24
33. Handbook on human nutritional requirements. Rome, FAO Nutr Stud No. 28, 1974
34. Hankin JH, Antonmattei JC: Survey of food service practices in nursing homes. Am J Public Health 50:1137, 1960
35. Henkin RI: Newer aspects of copper and zinc metabolism. In Mertz W, Cornatzer WE (eds): New Trace Elements in Nutrition. New York, M Dekker, 1971, pp 255–312
36. Irwin MI, Hegsted DM: A conspectus of research on protein requirements of man. J Nutr 101:385, 1971
37. Irwin MI, Hegsted DM: A conspectus of research on amino acid requirements of man. J Nutr 101:539, 1971
38. Jacobs A, Cavill IAJ, Hughes JNP: Erythrocyte transaminase activity. Effect of age, sex and vitamin B_6 supplementation. Am J Clin Nutr 21:502, 1968
39. Judge TV: The milieu intérieur and aging. In Brocklehurst JC (ed): Textbook of Geriatric Medicine and Gerontology. Edinburgh, Churchill Livingstone, 1973, pp 113–121
40. Kenny AD, Dacke CG: Parathyroid hormone and calcium metabolism. World Rev Nutr Diet 20: 231, 1975
41. Klevay LM: Coronary heart disease: the zinc/copper hypothesis. Am J Clin Nutr 28:764, 1975
42. LeBovit C, Baker DA: Food consumption and dietary levels of older households in Rochester, N.Y. Washington DC, Home Econ Res Rep No. 25, Agricultural Research Service, US Department of Agriculture, 1965
43. Levander OA: Selenium and chromium in human nutrition. J Am Diet Assoc 66:338, 1975
44. Mayer J: Obesity. In Goodhart RS, Shils ME (eds): Modern Nutrition in Health & Disease, 5th ed. Philadelphia, Lea & Febiger, 1973, pp 625–644
45. McDonald GW: The epidemiology of diabetes. In Ellenberg M, Rifkin H (eds): Diabetes Mellitus: Theory and Practice. New York, McGraw–Hill, 1970, pp 582–593
46. Mertz W, Roginski EE: Chromium metabolism, the glucose tolerance factor. In Mertz W, Cornatzer WE (eds): Newer Trace Elements in Nutrition. New York, M Dekker, 1971, pp 125–150
47. Mertz W, Toepfer EW, Roginski EE, Polansky MM: Present knowledge of the role of chromium. Fed Proc 33:2275, 1974
48. Miller WJ: Newer candidates for essential trace elements. Fed Proc 33:1747, 1974
49. Moriyama IM, Krueger DE, Stamler J (eds): Cardiovascular Disease in the United States. Cambridge, Harvard University Press, 1971, pp 63, 115–117
50. Munro HN: Protein requirements and metabolism in aging. In Carlson LA (ed): Nutrition in Old Age. Uppsala, Almqvist & Wiksell, 1972, pp 32–54
51. Murphy EW, Willis BW, Watt BK: Provisional tables on the zinc content of foods. J Am Diet Assoc 66:345, 1975

52. Neugarten BL: The roles we play. In Quality of Life: The Middle Years. National Congress by American Medical Association. Acton, MA, Publishing Sciences Group, 1974, pp 35–38
53. Nielsen FH, Ollerich DA: Nickel a new essential trace element. Fed Proc 33:1767, 1974
54. Nordin BEC: Metabolic Bone and Stone Disease. Baltimore, Williams & Wilkins, 1973, pp 30–34
55. Novak ER, Jones GS: Novak's Textbook of Gynecology. Baltimore, Williams & Wilkins, 1961, pp 118–120
56. Ohlson MA, Stearns G: Calcium intake of children and adults. Fed Proc 18: 1076, 1959
57. O'Kell RT, Elliott JR: Development of normal values for use in multitest biochemical screening of sera. Clin Chem 16:161, 1970
58. Painter NS: Pressures in the colon related to diverticular disease. Proc Roy Soc Med 63: suppl 144, 1970
59. Parker E: The Seven Ages of Woman. Baltimore, Johns Hopkins Press, 1960, pp 469–483
60. Peacock M, Gallagher JC, Nordin BEC: Action of 1 α-hydroxy vitamin D_3 on calcium absorption and bone resorption in man. Lancet 1:385, 1974
61. Pories WJ, Strain WH, Hsu JM, Woosley RL (eds): Clinical Applications of Zinc Metabolism. Springfield, Ill, CC Thomas, 1974
62. Preliminary Findings of the First Health and Nutrition Examination Survey, United States, 1971–1972: Dietary Intake and Biochemical Findings. DHEW No. (HRA) 74–1219-1. Rockville, MD, National Center for Health Statistics, 1974
63. Reed AH, Cannon DC, Winkelman JW, Bhasin YP, Henry RJ, Pileggi VJ: Estimation of normal ranges from a controlled sample survey. I. Sex- and age-related influence on the SMA 12/60 screening group of tests. Clin Chem 18:57, 1972
64. Report of a joint FAO/WHO Expert Group: Requirements of ascorbic acid, vitamin D, vitamin B_{12}, folate and iron. (WHO Tech Rep No. 452:5). Geneva, 1970
65. Report of a WHO Group of Experts: Nutritional anaemias. (WHO Tech Rep No. 503:5). Geneva, 1972
66. Report of a WHO Group of Experts: Trace elements in human nutrition. (WHO Tech Rep No. 532:5). Geneva, 1973
67. Rinzler SH: Primary prevention of coronary heart disease by diet. Bull NY Acad Med 44:936, 1968
68. Roberts LB: The normal ranges with statistical analysis for seventeen blood constituents. Clin Chim Acta 16:69, 1967
69. Schwarz K: Recent dietary trace element research exemplified by tin, fluorine and silicon. Fed Proc 33:1748, 1974
70. Scott ML: Role of selenium as an essential nutrient. In Mertz W, Cornatzer WE (eds): Newer Trace Elements in Nutrition. New York, M Dekker, 1971, p 86
71. Shapiro HR, Moore WT, Jorgensen H, Reid J, Epps CH, Whedon D: Osteoporosis, evaluation of diagnosis and therapy. Arch Intern Med 135:563, 1975
72. Shock NW: Physiological aspects of aging. J Am Diet Assoc 56:491, 1970
73. Skerlj B, Brozek J, Hunt EE Jr: Subcutaneous fat and age changes in body build and body form in women. Am J Phys Anthropol 11:577, 1953
74. Spencer H, Baladad J, Lewin I: The skeletal system; osteoporis. In Rossman I (ed): Clinical Geriatrics. Philadelphia, JB Lippincott, 1971, pp 285–289
75. Steinkamp RC, Cohen NL, Walsh HE: Resurvey of an aging population, fourteen year follow-up. The San Mateo Nutrition Study. J Am Diet Assoc 46:103, 1965
76. Strong JP, Eggen DA, Oalmann MC, Richards ML, Tracey RE: Pathology and epidemiology of atherosclerosis. J Am Diet Assoc 62:262, 1973
77. Taylor ES: Manual of Gynecology. Philadelphia, Lea & Febiger, 1952, pp 177–179
78. Ten-State Nutrition Survey 1968–1970, IV-Biochemical. DHEW No. (HSM)–72–8132, Atlanta, GA, Center for Disease Control, 1971

79. Ten-State Nutrition Survey 1968–1970, V-Dietary. DHEW No. (HSM)–72–8133, Atlanta, GA, Center for Disease Control, 1971

80. The role of fiber in the diet. Dairy Council Digest 46:1, 1975

81. Todhunter EN, House AF, VanderZwaag R: Food acceptance and food attitudes of the elderly as a basis for planning nutrition programs. Nashville, Tennessee Commission on Aging, 1974

82. Trowell H: Dietary fibre, ischaemic heart disease and diabetes mellitus. Proc Nutr Soc 32:151, 1973

83. Watkin DM: Nutrition for the aging and the aged. In Goodhart RS, Shils ME (eds): Modern Nutrition in Health and Disease, 5th ed. Philadelphia, Lea & Febiger, 1973, pp 681–710

84. Wessel JA, Ufer A, Van Huss WD, Cederquist D: Age trends of various components of body composition and functional characteristics in women aged 20–69 years. Ann NY Acad Sci 110:608, 1963

85. West KM: Prevention and therapy of diabetes mellitus. Nutr Rev 33:193, 1975

86. Whedon GD: Symposium comment. Osteoporosis. In Barzel US (ed): New York, Grune & Stratton, 1970, pp 266–272

87. Wilding P: Biochemical changes at the menopause. In Curry AS, Hewitt JV (eds): Biochemistry of Women: Clinical Concepts. Cleveland, CRC Press, 1974, pp 103–110

88. Wilding P, Rollason JG, Robinson D: Patterns of change for various biochemical constituents detected in well population screening. Clin Chim Acta 41:375, 1972

89. Wissler RW, Vesselinovitch D: Diet and experimental atherogenesis. In Chavez A, Bowiges H, Basta S (eds): Nutrition, Vol I. New York, S Karger, 1975, pp 333–339

90. Young CM, Blondin J, Tensuan R, Fryer JH: Body composition of "older" women. J Am Diet Assoc 43:344, 1963

91. Young CM, Blondin J, Tensuan R, Fryer JH: Body composition studies of "older" women, thirty to seventy years of age. Ann NY Acad Sci 110:589, 1963

92. Young CM, Martin MEK, Chihan M, McCarthy M, Mannielo MJ, Harmuth EH, Fryer JH: Body composition of young women. Some preliminary findings. J Am Diet Assoc 38:332, 1961

93. Young MM, Norden BEC: Effect of natural and artificial menopause on plasma and urinary calcium and phosphorus. Lancet 2: 118, 1967

Epilogue

Clinical Application of Nutrition in Perinatal Practice

Ronald A. Chez

In the preceding chapters of this book, an extraordinarily talented international roster of contributors has presented the current thinking in clinical nutrition and described the cutting edge of the current research in the area. I have been asked to present an epilog. I am unable to provide a denouement.

Our contributors have provided clinical tools for the practitioner that can be translated from the data that have been presented. Consider, as an illustrative example, a woman in early pregnancy seeking prenatal care in the United States. Her physician would—in addition to taking a complete history, physical examination, and screening laboratory examination—particularly emphasize her dietary history via a food intake frequency, a 24-hour recall, or a 3-day dietary history. The physician would search for and particularly emphasize those factors of weight, height, age, socioeconomic class, parity, medical aspects of previous pregnancies, current presence of chronic illness or infection, and the extent to which she uses cigarettes, alcohol, over-the-counter drugs, prescription drugs, and/or illicit drugs. During his continuing care for the gravida, the physician would particularly look for acetonuria, proteinuria, multiple pregnancy, and toxemia.

Because of his awareness of the need to gain information outside of his own realm of knowledge, the physician would be willing to consult outside sources: multi-media learning aids based on considerations of the ethnic, geographic, and cultural aspects of the patient; nutritionists; school teachers; social workers; government agencies; and perhaps, psychologists. He would recognize that the patient's wish to eat to appetite does not equate with free selection, but rather good nutrition requires guidance and education. And, if the patient were a teenager, the physician would have the insight to enhance her compliance by recommending such nutritious foods that may appear in the teenager's diet anyway, *i.e.*, ice cream, peanuts, and pizza.

The pregnancy might be monitored with ultrasound measurements of the biparietal and abdominal diameters during the second and third trimesters to provide information about appropriate fetal growth. The maternal urinary urea nitrogen/creatinine or urea nitrogen/total nitrogen ratios could be assayed to make a comment about the nutrition of this patient.

Because of this care, we would expect a maternal weight gain during gestation of about 24–28 pounds, the absence of functional or laboratory anemia, and a 3200+ g newborn.

If the patient wishes to breast feed, her continuing care would encompass the special needs of the lactating period.

Advice on family planning would review the various contraceptive modalities that are now available for a woman and her partner to use and would recognize that the oral contraceptive presently is the most effective reversible method both in theory and in use. The risks of its use would be weighed against the benefits. The risks would be evaluated with regard to both absolute and relative contraindications, with nutritional implications relating to vitamins and trace elements understood, and also with the knowledge that older age is the dominant statistical variant in the high-risk profiles relating oral contraceptives to the incidence of hypertension, glucose intolerance, and atherogenesis.

The physician would further recognize that in providing care, he has provided an entree for 2 patients, mother and conceptus, into a continual health care system. The nutrition of the newborn would be viewed with its potential effects on subsequent disease such as atherosclerosis, obesity, and diabetes mellitus. That is, he would comprehend that the child is in fact the father, or the mother, of the man.

What I have just described is *not* happening in this country. The question has to be, "Why not? What's wrong?" The easiest answer is that there is apathy and ignorance by both the patient and her physician.

First, the physician. For all intents and purposes, the physician's medical education is lacking. There is scant attention in our curricula to the aspects of nutrition. There are data that knowledge of clinical nutrition in medical centers is generally low except in those topics popular in the press. That is, the physician's knowledge is highly dependent upon nonmedical, nonprofessional literature.

Physicians are also buffeted with change as truth seekers discover today's magic substance. If he is old enough, the doctor remembers that pregnant women in the last 50 years were, at various times, treated with red meat only, then no meat, and then were starved. More recently, gravidas were restricted to an 18-pound weight gain with sodium restriction secondary to the fear of overnutrition and the belief that edema was the harbinger of toxemia. Today, the "in" thing is to let the patient gain between 24–28 pounds and salt her high protein food to taste. We now "know" that edema is a normal physiologic accompaniment of pregnancy, as is glucosuria, and that A and D vitamin overdosage can damage the fetus.

All of these comments are made with the full knowledge that the information presented to us here, as in the past, has been by the most sincere, dedicated, competent, and well-intentioned scientists. They are made as a plea that all of us who are in science not take ourselves too seriously, and not lose our sense of humor, perspective, or proportion.

The physician is also accosted by the hard sell for lactation and breast feeding. One problem is that otherwise objective scientists seem unable to discuss this subject without emotion and bias. There are benefits for the newborn from breast milk. Perhaps one of the benefits is that the newborn will not be overfed, although it is difficult to use that terminology when *both* length and body mass are increased in bottle-fed babies. A disadvantage of lactation is that the patient is denied the use of the most effective reversible contraceptive agent we have, the combination pill. Furthermore, lactation also insures that those drugs and adverse substrates that were crossing from the mother through the placenta to the fetus now will continue to be received by the newborn through her breast milk.

Given that the physician is knowledgeable and a seeker after the truth, what diagnostic tools can he apply to his patient? If he wishes to provide an accurate clinical assessment of nutrition intake, the diet history from a 24-hour recall or a 3-day average suffers from lack of validity. Clues in the physical examination can be extremely subtle and, therefore, easily missed. There are no clear-cut assays to run on maternal urine or blood or amniotic fluid. Even the scale that we use to weigh people cannot differentiate between normal fluid retention and excess fat retention.

From the point of view of diagnosis, there remain the uncertainties of what truly constitutes deprivation, what is anemia, what is normal variability, and what is the range of physiologic change? We do not know what is the appropriate use of the RDA for the individual patient. The RDA is based on data which allow very different interpretations by very equivalent and competent judges. It is set at a level two standard deviations above the estimated mean requirement and therefore is not significant for all women throughout all age groups with all degrees of physical activity.

Given that a diagnosis of malnutrition can be made, then what is the treatment? The treatment is food! Too often, that is something not understood. But even with food treatment in the antepartum period, there is a strong suggestion that we are too late because we are not in the preconceptual period. The benefits are further diminished if we wait until after the first trimester into the second trimester. Then, there is the issue, do we use proteins or do we use calories? And then what route?—maternal oral, maternal intravascular, or intraamniotic? If the latter, what about excess osmolality and the development of excess fetal blood and tissue levels with unknown dangers?

Can the physician expect help from the team? Nutritionists are frequently overburdened with administrative work and may not be encouraged to practice or ask research questions. There are a surfeit of reading learning aids, but some otherwise excellent booklets use measures of ounces and grams instead of portion sizes. Visual aids are scant, and a good movie is not yet available. Our government, as part of the team, sometimes seems to emphasize underdeveloped countries in the world and not the underdeveloped counties in the United States. There are benefits from the United States Department of Agriculture programs. The Nutrition Bill is now law. And although it is easy to carp at the administrative procedures they entail, the deficiencies of those programs are no different than they would be with any bureaucratic program—whether it be state, local or federal governments or a large corporation. However, it is also true that we do not have a national policy on maternal health and nutrition at this time.

Patients are also members of the therapeutic team. Our patient has very personal tastes that have been cultivated by ethnic, cultural, and economic considerations. She is exposed constantly to short-order cooking, prepackaged foods, and precooked meals. She recognizes, perhaps on a subliminal level, that nutrition is merely a function of her total well being, and she has a specific priority for it. That priority competes with rent, clothing, transportation, entertainment, and other elements of life. She is also a member of a nuclear family and usually does not eat alone. Rather, her family may include a child, an adolescent, a husband, and sometimes a parent or grandparent. Therefore, whatever diet she consumes should have equivalency and be acceptable to all in that wide range of age and sex. Our patient is, but should not be, confronted with aid which is sporadic because it is given as a bolus rather than a long-term infusion. And so often our aid, if it is food, is divorced from the spectrum of help that is required for total care. This approach denies the plea: "Give me a fish, I eat for a day. Teach me to fish, I eat for a lifetime."

And what about the research that is going on in this area? There can be no doubt of its extremely high caliber use of scientific method. But there are problems. There is the difficulty in defining a normal female, the difficulty in defining physiologic indices, and the difficulty in defining pharmacologic amounts versus physiologic amounts when a system is stressed or challenged. Clinical obstetrics teaches that nature does not always know best, but nature does offer clues. The high incidence in apparently normal women of first trimester nausea and vomiting, constipation, heartburn, leg cramps, and edema suggests evolutionary benefit that requires deciphering. There are also uncertainties in extrapolating from species to species because of length of gestation, type of placenta, litter size, ratio of conceptus to total maternal weight, type of normal diet, and functional capability of the newborn.

What is the appropriate role of lactation in our population? It does seem that if two-thirds to three-fourths of our patients choose not to breast-feed, perhaps they may know something we do not know. We could listen to our patients before we go ahead and impose our particular prejudices. Certainly it is unfair that our clinical approach is to attempt to imbue women with guilt for not breast-feeding their infants.

What about oral contraceptives? Statistical studies are important, but they must be put into perspective because all of us care for patients as individuals, not as large groups. The perspective of any prescription is the risk/benefit ratio for that woman. We have to differentiate between casual and causal associations. The relative ubiquity of the pill—30% of the women in the reproductive years in the United States use the combination pill—means that pill users could constitute one-third of the women in any group in which some abnormality is found. We must be cautious so that before we go ahead and replace or limit the use of the pill to any great extent we have something which is as efficacious with which to replace it. This admonition seems particularly pertinent since men, for the most part, are the ones who prescribe the contraceptive method and men, for the most part, do not assume responsibility for the use of a contraceptive method.

Finally, there is the problem of the subject itself—nutrition. Somehow it lacks the pizazz and the glamor that we so often find with other topics—such as sex. About 10 years ago some doctors started listening and began to understand their patient's feelings of inadequacies with their sexuality. They were also introspective enough to understand their own personal feelings of inadequacies in this area. These doctors, through effective lobbying, got sexuality on to the medical curriculum, admittedly often using sensationalism to do so. Raw sex was their magic substance, and they managed to produce a nice appropriate blend of panic and interest which resulted in the granting of resources, time, and money. Once they got their initial message across, they settled down, achieved respectability, and now are concentrating on getting their real message across—that sex is merely one facet of interpersonal relationships and can reflect the rest of the interpersonal relationship. It does not stand alone. Similarly, food is only one facet of total well being; good nutrition does not stand alone.

When I went to medical school more than 20 years ago, the first time we learned about pregnancy was at 6 weeks' gestation. It is now known that sex comes first. Sex has had its day and now it is pregnancy's turn. Now is the chance for nutrition in the perinatal period to have its day. Least you disagree too much with my analogy to sex, please remember that zinc, today's magic substance, and food are both four-letter words.